ISSUES IN AGING AND VISION

ALBERTA L. ORR

ISSUES IN AGING AND VISION

A Curriculum for University Programs and In-Service Training

ALBERTA L. ORR

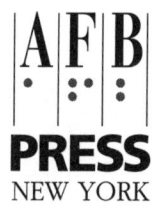

AFB PRESS
NEW YORK

Issues in Aging and Vision: A Curriculum for University Programs and In-Service Training, is copyright © 1998 by AFB Press, American Foundation for the Blind.

All rights reserved. No part of this work may be reproduced or transmitted in any form or by any means, electronic or mechanical, including photocopying and recording, or by any information storage or retrieval system, except as may be expressly permitted by the 1976 Copyright Act, or in writing from the publisher. Requests for permission should be addressed in writing to AFB Press, American Foundation for the Blind, 11 Penn Plaza, Suite 300, New York, NY 10001.

Printed in the United States of America.

Library of Congress Cataloging-in-Publication Data
Orr, Alberta L., 1950-
 Issues in aging and vision: a curriculum for university programs and in-service training / Alberta L. Orr.
     p. cm.
 Includes bibliographical references.
 ISBN 0-89128-947-X
 1. Visually handicapped aged—Rehabilitation—Study and teaching. 2. Vision disorders in old age—Study and teaching. I. Title.
HV 1597.5.O79 1998
362.4'1'0846—dc21   98-6543
                                                                                                 CIP

This project was made possible by a grant from the National Institute on Disability and Rehabilitation Research, U.S. Department of Education, No. H133G30053.

Contents

	FOREWORD	vii
	PREFACE	ix
	ACKNOWLEDGMENTS	xi
	INTRODUCTION	xiii
MODULE 1.	The Demographics of Aging and Vision Loss: Implications for Service Delivery	1
MODULE 2.	The Aging Eye: Age-Related Eye Conditions and Their Functional Implications	32
MODULE 3.	The Psychosocial Aspects of Aging and Vision Loss: Impact on the Older Person, Family Members, and the Family Unit	84
MODULE 4.	Community-Based Services for Older Persons Who Are Blind or Visually Impaired	107
MODULE 5.	Improving Access to Vision Rehabilitation and Support Services	142
MODULE 6.	Trends and Issues in Vision-Related Rehabilitation Services	167

MODULE 7. Building Effective Partnerships Between the Aging Network and the Vision Rehabilitation Field **198**

GLOSSARY **215**

ABOUT THE AUTHOR **223**

Foreword

At the end of the twentieth century, the phrase "the graying of America" has already become something of a cliche. We all know that our population is living longer. Yet, as *Issues in Aging and Vision* points out, the number of older people in the U.S. population is expected to double between now and 2030, when one person in five will be age 65 or older.

Because the incidence of vision loss increases sharply with age, age-related visual impairment is an increasing concern for all of us, and one whose significance will continue to grow. It is essential, therefore, that anyone who works with older people be conscious of the issues that confront individuals who lose their vision at an advanced age, aware of the signs of vision loss, and knowledgeable about helping clients get the vision-related services they need. Professionals and service providers in a variety of areas will find that this unique curriculum will answer their own needs in this regard. It provides all the materials a teacher or trainer requires, whether it be for presenting a brief workshop or teaching an entire university course on aging and vision. It is also a valuable reference tool.

But even beyond these important practical uses, *Issues in Aging and Vision* is intended to be a consciousness raiser for professionals in both the fields of aging and vision rehabilitation alike. As these fields increasingly intersect, it is critical that service providers work together across professional boundaries to help their mutual clients. In an era in which funding for services is shrinking, professional collaboration and advocacy is more important than ever in maintaining access to the services that older people who are blind or visually impaired need.

The American Foundation for the Blind is proud to publish this ground-breaking work, the result of a four-year project, and thereby contribute to that critical collaboration.

Carl R. Augusto
President
American Foundation for the Blind

Preface

When I was in graduate school, a particularly wise professor of mine was fond of saying that when he taught medical students and other health personnel, he admonished them to pay close attention because what he was about to tell them would make not only their patients' lives, but their own, easier and better. What he meant, of course, was that the effective, practical advice about how to care for the often complex and difficult problems presented by older patients would make these incipient practitioners more successful, more appreciated, and, therefore, more satisfied with their work. Work satisfaction, he knew, came from doing a good job, which in the field of aging often means solving the thorniest of problems.

Although gerontology has learned much in the last 25 years about the aging process and how to make later life a better time, much of what we know still is not being transmitted to the next generation of gerontological and geriatric practitioners. We can blame this failure on (a) an overloaded curriculum—never has there been so much to know; (b) training program designs that lag behind the exploding knowledge curve; or (c) faculty and in-service coordinators who are well-intentioned but overburdened and unable to incorporate the latest advances on every topic related to aging. The best answer and most likely explanation is (d) all of the above. Busy faculty and busy training planners simply are being overwhelmed with new information and new claims on their curricula.

So, here is one more claim: vision problems of older people. All of us in the field of aging acknowledge the importance of knowing about sensory losses, but unless we teach a course in the health field, we often give only cursory attention to the specific problems and how to address them. Alberta Orr, one of the most recognized names in the field of aging and vision, is determined to change our teaching behavior with this new book published by AFB Press. She makes a powerful and compelling case for inclusion of more information about vision problems—and solutions—in the modern curriculum on aging. Read even the Introduction, and you will be convinced of the significance and centrality of vision in an aging society.

But if you read on, you will find that this is a sound and user-friendly volume. Orr knows her audience well. She and her colleague, Dr. Nora Griffin-Shirley, prepared for this volume by doing a careful study of gerontologists and their academic programs, determining what they knew about vision and vision problems and what kinds of information they were likely to use in their courses. Armed with this insight, Orr has crafted a state-of-the-art curriculum designed with the busy gerontology faculty member in mind. One can assign those modules that fit best in the course or courses one teaches and simply read the others to become quite knowledgeable about this important area of our field.

We are in Alberta Orr's debt for the inventive yet careful way she has prepared this material for our use. I have a notion that, if we listen to her and incorporate even some of her information and ideas into our lectures and readings, we will make our students better at what they are training to do, and that will make them happier in their jobs and more grateful to us for having taught them well.

Frank J. Whittington, Ph.D.
Professor of Sociology
Director, Gerontology Center
Georgia State University
Atlanta, Georgia

Acknowledgments

The author wishes to thank Priscilla Rogers of Aging Futures, Mooresburg, TN, and Maureen Duffy, Director, Master of Science Program in Rehabilitation Teaching, Pennsylvania College of Optometry, Philadelphia, for their expert contributions in reviewing this curriculum. A special note of thanks is also extended to Dr. Alfred A. Rosenbloom, Director, Low Vision Service, The Chicago Lighthouse for the Blind and Visually Impaired, for his review of the module on low vision. Thanks are also due to all the university faculty who reviewed and commented on many versions of the curriculum, as well as to university faculty and gerontology program alumni who participated in the initial study to determine the level of interest in a curriculum within university programs providing course work on aging throughout the country.

The author also wishes to thank the National Institute on Disability and Rehabilitation Research, U.S. Department of Education, for the funding that supported the effort to investigate the need for and development of this curriculum and its accompanying video, *Profiles in Aging and Vision*.

Introduction

This seven-module curriculum on aging and vision loss has been developed by the American Foundation for the Blind (AFB) for use in university gerontology programs, in-service training programs, and related courses throughout the country. The purpose of this curriculum is to prepare current and future service providers, planners, and administrators to improve the delivery of vision-related rehabilitation services and home- and community-based long-term services to older individuals who are experiencing vision loss. The curriculum's goal is to heighten readers' awareness of the growing population of older Americans experiencing age-related vision loss and the continued growth of this population in the next millennium. Its intent is to ensure that older visually impaired persons have access to the services they need to continue living as independently and productively as possible, for as long as possible, in their own homes and communities.

The need for the curriculum is based on several factors. Already, nearly 5 million older Americans experience vision loss that is severe enough to interfere with their ability to carry out routine daily tasks (see Module 1). The vast majority are still living in their own homes and communities, but approximately 364,000 older visually impaired persons are in nursing-home settings (Schmeidler

& Halfmann, 1998). The growth in this group is associated with the burgeoning population of older Americans who are living longer and encountering physical conditions and health problems associated with the aging process.

Four of the five leading causes of vision loss in the United States are age related. The population of older persons who are severely visually impaired is expected to double by the year 2030, when the last cohort of the baby boom generation reaches its senior years; it is already as large as the number of older people with Alzheimer's disease. Yet service providers who encounter older clients who are visually impaired often feel unprepared to serve these clients most effectively. They may feel that their knowledge base, experience, and skills in this area are limited, and they are likely to be unfamiliar with the life issues specific to age-related vision loss, the impact of vision loss on routine functioning, and the resources available to ameliorate the effects of vision loss. Thus, it is becoming increasingly crucial to prepare students for work with this target population.

Background

Gerontologists at AFB, along with members of a national advisory committee on aging, began talking about the need to develop a curriculum on aging and vision loss to educate professionals in the field of aging in the late 1980s. According to Denton (1990), most professionals working in the field of aging never had the opportunity for any formal education or training in vision loss and, therefore, they were not prepared to work effectively with this growing population. Researchers such as Rogers and Long (1991) and Orr (1991) pointed to the lack of and need for gerontological training programs in this area. Through an innovation grant from the National Institute on Disability and Rehabilitation Research (NIDRR) of the U.S. Department of Education, AFB conducted a project to research, develop, and disseminate guidelines for a competency-based curriculum for institutions of higher education that offer course work in gerontology (Griffin-Shirley & Orr, 1993).

To determine the climate nationally for a curriculum on aging and vision, AFB conducted a formal investigation during the 1991-92 academic year. The investigation included national surveys of university gerontology programs, individual faculty members, and alumni to determine the state of the art in curriculum content on aging and vision loss in university gerontology programs. The results indicated that limited curriculum content existed on vision loss topics beyond the normal vision changes associated with aging and that there was broad interest in infusing content on aging and vision loss into existing university curricula. Many faculty members who were surveyed indicated both a lack of awareness about the population of older people who are visually impaired and a need for resources on aging and vision loss. Incorporating a complete new course on aging and vision into gerontology programs was seen as less feasible, however, particularly in a time of economic difficulty, when many gerontology programs are struggling to stay alive on campuses, to maintain their separate identity as a discipline or as an interdisciplinary program, and not to be subsumed within another department (Griffin-Shirley & Orr, 1993). The results of this research led to a three-year field-initiated research grant from NIDRR to develop, test, and publish this curriculum and its accompanying video, *Profiles in Aging and Vision*.

Since the initial surveys were conducted, considerable change has taken place that has prepared the gerontology community for this curriculum. A growing number of people, both professionals and the general public, are becoming increasingly aware of the prevalence of age-related vision loss and its impact on family life. More individuals and their families, especially the parents of today's baby boomers, are experiencing firsthand the effects of age-related eye conditions. The media have recognized the need for more information, and eye conditions such as macular degeneration have received a considerable degree of media attention.

Uses for the Curriculum

Issues in Aging and Vision was originally developed to address the need for information on aging and vision loss at the master's degree level, specifically in university gerontology programs. As the curriculum developers and a panel of experts developed the guidelines for the development of the curriculum content, it became clear that the curriculum would be applicable across many professional disciplines and at various levels of academic education and in-service training. The use of the curriculum will vary from application to

INTRODUCTION

application at the various levels of education and training, in regard to the depth of the content covered, variations in teaching methods, and the amount of time allocated for coverage of topics dealing with aging and vision loss.

University gerontology programs range from specific programs offering degrees in gerontology to interdisciplinary degree programs in gerontology to degree programs in other professional disciplines with concentrations in aging. Among these other disciplines are social work, occupational therapy, physical therapy, nursing, counseling, and family studies. Universities with programs in aging may offer a degree, certificate, minor, concentration, specialization, emphasis, or track in aging; these may be research or clinical programs in gerontology, geriatrics, or aging studies.

To maximize the use of the curriculum among gerontology faculty, it has been designed in modules so that it can be adopted and taught in its entirety, by individual module, or by a combination of modules as appropriate to the course content and the time available. The modules are relevant for both academic and applied or professional programs.

The curriculum also can be used for in-service training or continuing education for service providers who are already working in the aging field but who have not had the opportunity to develop a knowledge base in the issues of aging and age-related vision loss. Service providers in the field of vision rehabilitation routinely conduct in-service training for professionals in the aging network and in allied health care fields to heighten levels of awareness about the subpopulation of older visually impaired people, the issues they confront, and the services available in the vision rehabilitation field. The curriculum modules also can serve to complement already established training materials or to enable professionals at an agency that has not yet developed in-service training materials to get started. And, increasingly, public and private agencies serving people who are blind or visually impaired and local Area Agencies on Aging are working together to provide cross-training between the two service delivery systems to educate each other about available services and how the services available through each system can complement and build on each other, so that older consumers can obtain the comprehensive package of services they need from an array of professional disciplines.

Content of the Curriculum

The content of the curriculum represents the results of the national surveys conducted, as well as input from the project's advisory committee and its panel of experts who participated in a working group on curriculum development. The seven modules are as follows:

1. The Demographics of Aging and Vision Loss: Implications for Service Delivery
2. The Aging Eye: Age-Related Eye Conditions and Their Functional Implications
3. The Psychosocial Aspects of Aging and Vision Loss: Impact on the Older Person, Family Members, and the Family Unit
4. Community-Based Services for Older Persons Who Are Blind or Visually Impaired
5. Improving Access to Vision Rehabilitation and Support Services
6. Trends and Issues in Vision-Related Rehabilitation Services
7. Building Effective Partnerships Between the Aging Network and the Vision Rehabilitation Field

This curriculum has been designed to be as flexible as possible. The modules can be used in any of a variety of ways to develop an entirely new course on aging and age-related vision loss or to enhance ongoing course work and degree programs in gerontology, without extensive preparation on the part of faculty. Thus, if a full course is not feasible, entire modules or portions of modules can be integrated into existing courses. In addition, various portions of each module can be selected to develop a continuing education course on the issues and service needs regarding aging and age-related vision loss.

For example, Module 2, "The Aging Eye," could easily be incorporated into courses such as the Biology of Aging or the Physiology of Aging, which typically cover only normal age-related changes in the eye, or into courses on Health and Aging or Aging and Disabilities. A course such as Aging and Disabilities would also logically incorporate Module 3, "The Psychosocial Aspects of Aging and Vision Loss," to help students become familiar with the life issues and circumstances resulting from an impairment or compounding impairments. Module 3 could also easily be incorporated into a course on the Psychology of Aging, the Social Psychology of Aging and Disability, or other courses covering the psychosocial aspects of aging. A course on Aging and Social Policy could incorporate information in Modules 4 and 5 about the Rehabilitation Act along with discussion of the Older Americans Act and other significant legislation affecting older Americans. Many undergraduate gerontology programs could include portions of Modules 2, 3, and 4 in their Introduction to Aging courses.

The curriculum would also be useful in courses in disability studies or developmental disabilities, which are offered more frequently since the passage of the Americans with Disabilities Act. Just as the professionals in the aging network need to give attention to disability, including aging with a lifelong disability and onset of disability late in life, leaders in the disability arena need to turn their attention to the aging population and its increasing experience with various forms of functional impairment and disabling conditions.

It is suggested that a minimum of 2 hours be spent on each module in order for students to gain a basic familiarity with the key issues, service needs, and availability of services for the aging visually impaired population. The entire curriculum can be covered in approximately 7 sessions, each 2 to 3 hours in length. If time permits, the course could more effectively be taught in 14 or 15 sessions, with 2 sessions devoted to each module. A 15-session course would provide time to cover essential information and to permit students to participate in hands-on, experiential learning activities, such as small-group brainstorming sessions, role playing, guest speakers, demonstrations, and visits to vision rehabilitation agencies.

The students taking the courses in which this curriculum is utilized will range from those in graduate, undergraduate, or associate degree programs to those participating in gerontology certificate programs at various levels (including post-master's certificate programs) and continuing education courses. In addition, portions of the curriculum will be used for in-service training sessions for service providers representing many professional disciplines who are already working in the aging or vision rehabilitation field who may not have had the opportunity for such course work prior to their employment.

Learning Objectives

The curriculum is based on the needs of professionals who work with older persons who are experiencing vision loss or who are blind or visually impaired. Because vision loss is an unaddressed or underaddressed topic in gerontological education, many gerontology professionals feel unprepared to work with older visually impaired persons and less able to ensure that their clients' vision-related service needs are being met. This curriculum is designed to empower current and future workers in the field of aging by providing information about the life crisis issues of this target population. Thus, the purpose of this curriculum is to translate the needs of potential students into curriculum objectives (Knowles, 1986). These objectives specify the changes in the behavior patterns of students or workers in response to older consumers who are blind or visually impaired that are expected to result from the learning to be acquired through the seven curriculum modules (Tyler, 1952).

The range of curriculum content and the learner objectives have been chosen to equip professionals in the field of aging with the knowledge base and the skills to respond effectively to this consumer group. Students will acquire an understanding of the older visually impaired person within several contexts, including the aging process itself and the familial context, and within the context of the aging and vision rehabilitation service delivery systems. They also will learn how the two fields must work together to meet the holistic needs of older individuals—their psychological adjustment and their physical and psychological well-being.

The primary learning objectives for the seven-module curriculum are as follows:

Module 1. Students will be able to describe the growth in the population of older persons experiencing age-related vision loss within the context of an aging society and the importance of having accurate demographic data in order to plan, advocate for, and deliver targeted services.

Students will be exposed to demographic data about the aging population and the prevalence of vision loss among this group. This module will help students understand the implications of this data for available services and service delivery models and methods and the need for public policies to respond to these demographic trends.

Module 2. Students will be able to describe normal age-related functional vision changes, the eye conditions associated with aging, the types of vision loss associated with each eye condition, and the functional implications of each condition.

These eye conditions include macular degeneration, glaucoma, diabetic retinopathy, and cataracts. This knowledge base will help workers understand the type of vision loss experienced by an older person with one of these eye conditions, how it affects daily functioning, its prognosis, and whether any medical treatment is available to correct vision or prevent further deterioration of vision.

Module 3. Students will be able to describe the impact of vision loss on the older person, on individual family members, particularly spouses and adult children, and on the family unit as a whole.

This module will enable students to understand the physical and psychological losses associated with vision loss, issues along the independence-dependence continuum and how they affect the older individual and his or her family members, as well as the changes in roles and reactions among family members and significant others in response to the onset of vision loss.

Module 4. Students will be able to describe the workings of the vision rehabilitation system as well as the vision-related services available to address the needs of older persons experiencing vision loss.

The module will provide students with an understanding of the structure of the service delivery system, the specific vision-related rehabilitation services that enable people who are blind or visually impaired to continue to function independently, and the specialized vision professionals who provide these services.

Module 5. Students will demonstrate the ability to identify community resources, the structure of the vision rehabilitation service delivery system, and the services available to ameliorate the impact of vision loss on older visually impaired persons and their family members.

Students will learn about the range of services that are available to the older person experiencing vision loss and that can maximize independent functioning while providing appropriate support. Specific information will include eligibility criteria, funding levels, and the referral process, in order to ensure that older visually impaired persons are served effectively and do not "fall between the cracks" in the referral process between the aging and vision-related service delivery systems.

Module 6. Students will be able to describe current issues and trends in delivery of vision-related rehabilitation services to older people experiencing age-related vision loss.

Students will learn about innovative methods of service delivery in the field of vision rehabilitation, as well as current issues such as the ongoing need for increased funding for vision-related services targeted specifically for older people; debates over moving vision rehabilitation services into the health care arena and the issues related to third-party reimbursement of vision-related services; and the need for advocacy in the public policy arena.

Module 7. Students will be able to describe the importance of collaboration between the aging and vision fields and the skills needed to build networks and partnerships between the vision and the aging service delivery systems to serve older visually impaired clients more comprehensively, efficiently, and effectively.

This module will teach students that older persons who are blind or visually impaired are consumers of both the aging and the vision rehabilitation service delivery systems and that collaborative planning and service delivery between these two fields on behalf of this population is crucial to effective and comprehensive rehabilitation and adjustment to vision loss.

Sequence of the Modules

According to Knowles (1972), the sequence of a curriculum is important in timing learning to coincide with learners' developmental tasks and readiness to learn. The sequence of the material in this curriculum takes into consideration Knowles' andragogical design for learning, which includes (1) setting a climate, (2) diagnosing needs, (3) formulating program objectives, (4) planning a sequential design of learning activities, (5) conducting the learning experiences and enhancing the learning, (6) carrying out mutual planning and implementation of the learning process, and (7) evaluating the learning. (It should be noted that the andragogical approach to teaching and learning with adults is applied to all aspects of vision-related rehabilitation services for adults who are blind or visually impaired.)

When following the entire curriculum, the learner is first immersed in the biological and factual aspects of vision loss, then builds on the understanding of feelings and reactions to vision loss, and finally proceeds to problem solving (which is an important aspect of the adult learner's orientation to learning) to ensure the provision of comprehensive services. Thus, when the curriculum is used in its entirety, the specified sequence allows students to build their knowledge base in each content area.

Structure of the Modules

In addition to the curriculum content for each module, the modules also include the following:

- an introduction and summary
- a list of topics covered
- a set of learner objectives
- references cited
- recommended teaching methods
- resources, including
    - recommended readings
    - additional readings for more in-depth exploration of the content
    - other resources for additional information and exploration of the topics
- for most modules, fact sheets or handouts for students
- in some cases, an appendix

The learner objectives are provided to give faculty members or trainers the essential points needed by the learner. They have been kept simple and brief, and faculty members can add to them as needed.

The suggested teaching methods were developed to offer professionals using the curriculum a variety of alternatives and are based on the methods used to teach courses on aging and vision loss within the master's degree programs in the vision rehabilitation field in orientation and mobility and rehabilitation teaching. An overview of the methods suggested in the modules appears later in this introduction. Because the amount of time available in the classroom can determine the use of various teaching methods, some of the suggestions can be used as assignments. For example, students can work in small groups to brainstorm on a topic between class sessions, rather than in class; or individuals or small groups may arrange to visit a vision rehabilitation agency or low vision clinic for a required project rather than during a class session.

The recommended readings listed are those most closely associated with the content included in the curriculum and can be used prior to and after class time devoted to learning about vision loss.

The additional readings include more in-depth or technical references that can be used by students in preparation for writing required papers.

A variety of other information is provided in the resource sections, including additional reference materials, relevant organizations to contact, and sources for related products and services. These resources can be used in a variety of ways. These sections can be especially useful as materials to distribute to participants in in-service training sessions. The fact sheets are also designed to be copied and used as handouts. Some are written as resources for service providers and others are designed specifically for distribution to older visually impaired individuals and their family members.

Profiles in Aging and Vision: The Video

The curriculum is accompanied by a 30-minute instructional videotape, *Profiles in Aging and Vision.* The video is designed to be used as an overview of the curriculum's topics and as an introduction to the curriculum for faculty using the complete curriculum or any of the modules or combinations thereof. Professionals, older individuals who have experienced age-related vision loss, and their family members describe the vision-related rehabilitation services available and the difference that these services can make in the lives of older people. Older people and their family members relate their reactions to the onset of vision loss late in life, and explain how professionals in the vision rehabilitation field can provide instruction in adaptive techniques and the use of adaptive devices so that older people who lose their vision can continue to live productive, independent, and satisfying lives.

Recommended Teaching Methods

As noted, the topics covered in this curriculum on aging and vision lend themselves to a variety of teaching methods. Suggestions are made in each module about the most appropriate methods for that material. These can be adapted depending on the time available.

Lecture

The lecture method is particularly important in teaching a topic that is relatively new to most students and in which the presentation of content is essential.

Group Discussions

Active participation on the part of the learner is a primary condition of learning (Perlman, 1951). Opportunities for discussion in both small groups and with the entire class allow learners to share experiences regarding loss in general and vision loss specifically from both a professional and a personal context. Group participation allows students within an andragogical perspective to demonstrate and experience that they, too, are resource persons within the teaching and learning context (Knowles, 1972).

Brainstorming Sessions

Brainstorming sessions are useful for helping students identify certain areas of knowledge from their own personal or prior work experience. Before presenting the content of Modules 4, 5, and 6 involving specific services and resources, for example, it can be useful to organize students into small groups to see if they can identify on their own what kinds of services people will need when they lose vision. It is also an important technique for Module 3, in which students can brainstorm about the impact of vision loss on older individuals from either personal or professional experience.

Logs or Journals

Faculty may want to request that students keep a log or a journal during the course of the training. Germain (1991) proposed the log or journal as an effective means of helping students integrate content knowledge and their personal responses to that learning. Use of a log can help students integrate the learning, particularly as it relates to the impact of vision loss on the older person, their own feelings about the aging process, the physiological and psychological issues related to independent functioning throughout the aging process, and issues related to their own parents and their own roles as current or future caregivers.

Role Playing

Role playing is also an important learning method for students of this curriculum. Role playing allows students to examine and critique the nuances of worker-client involvement (Swell, 1968). In this curriculum, role playing is generally used after lecture material has been presented and after small-group brainstorming has been completed, when students have gained enough knowledge and understanding of the material to portray the roles. Role playing should be used discriminately as the teacher observes the extent of its success and usefulness within the dynamics of each class.

Guest Speakers and Field Visits

Because the course content may be new to many of those who will be teaching the curriculum, it may be useful to call upon professionals in the community to share their expertise with faculty and students. For example, a low vision specialist could describe the benefits of low vision services and devices, or someone from a state rehabilitation agency might describe how the older consumer becomes eligible for vision-related rehabilitation services. Visiting an agency can also be an invaluable experience for students. Field visits can be scheduled beyond course hours, either as a required or as an optional learning experience to expand the time available within the course hours.

Demonstrations, Activities, and Exercises

Because much of this curriculum will be new to most students, it is important for the teacher to include demonstrations, hands-on activities, and experiential exercises. For example, the teacher may initiate opportunities for students to examine optical and nonoptical adaptive devices, or to understand how people see with various eye conditions by trying on eyeglasses that simulate these conditions.

Evaluation of Students' Learning

Faculty members can evaluate their own knowledge base as well as that of students by using the pretest included at the end of this introduction. Responses to this pretest will provide the instructor with students' basic perceptions about the impact of vision loss on the older person prior to the course work. Students can complete the same instrument as a posttest to determine changes in their perceptions and attitudes and to evaluate learning.

Providing a Context

As teachers present the material contained in these modules, it will be important for them to provide a context for vision loss, making clear that the impact is great, that adjustment is a process, that certain supports or lack of supports enhance or inhibit the process, and that older visually impaired persons need not be viewed as completely dependent on the formal service delivery system or on the informal network of caregivers. This understanding, along with the knowledge gained through this curriculum, will enable and empower service providers in the field of aging to assist older visually impaired clients and thus empower them to seek the services they need. Through this curriculum content, service providers will be more prepared to

- understand the life circumstances of an older person who is losing vision;
- know what services are available within the vision rehabilitation arena for older persons; and
- understand their responsibility not just to refer older visually impaired clients to the vision rehabilitation system, but to serve them as mutual clients of both the aging and vision service delivery systems.

References

Denton, D. R. (1990). *Caring for an aging society: Issues and strategies for gerontological education.* Atlanta: Southern Regional Education Board.

Germain, C. B. (1991). An instructor's story about students' life stories. In R. R. Middleman & G. G. Wood (Eds.), *Teaching secrets: The technology in social work education* (pp. 3–13). Binghamton, NY: Haworth Press.

Griffin-Shirley, N., & Orr, A. L. (1993). *Aging and vision loss: Guidelines for an innovative personnel preparation curriculum in gerontology.* Final Report to the National Institute on Disability and Rehabilitation Research (No. H133C10187). Washington, DC: U.S. Department of Education.

Knowles, M. S. (1972). Innovations in teaching styles and approaches based upon adult learning. *Journal of Education for Social Work, 8*(2), 32–39.

Knowles, M. S. (1986). *The modern practice of adult education.* New York: Adult Education Co.

Orr, A. L. (1991). The psychosocial aspects of aging and vision. In N. Weber (Ed.), *Vision and aging: Issues in social work practice* (pp. 1–14). Binghamton, NY: Haworth Press.

Perlman, H. (1951). The lecture as a method in teaching casework. *Social Service Review, 25*(1), 19–32.

Rogers, P., & Long, R. (1991). The challenge of establishing a national service delivery program for older blind persons. *Journal of Gerontological Social Work, 17*(3/4), 153–164.

Schmeidler, E., & Halfmann, D. (1998). Vision of nursing home residents; expected years of healthy life; and risk factors for adolescents. Demographics Update. *Journal of Visual Impairment & Blindness, 92*(3), 221–224.

Swell, L. (1968). Role playing in the context of learning theory in casework. *Journal of Education for Social Work, 4*(1).

Tyler, R. (1952, April). Distinctive attributes of education for the profession. *Social Work Journal.*

Aging and Age-Related Vision Loss Pretest

Indicate whether the statement is true (T) or false (F) in the space provided:

_____ Older visually impaired persons accept gradually deteriorating vision loss as a natural part of the aging process and therefore do not typically seek services to ameliorate its impact.

_____ Older persons experiencing vision loss and their family members need to seriously consider nursing home placement.

_____ Most older visually impaired persons can continue to live independently and require no assistance from anyone.

_____ There are no rehabilitation services available for older people who lose their vision, so they must be cared for by their family members.

_____ Fewer than a million older persons in the United States are blind or visually impaired.

_____ Vision loss is one of the most highly feared impairments among older persons, and within the general population as well.

_____ Older visually impaired persons can learn to use a white cane and travel independently throughout their community.

_____ Persons in their late 50s or 60s who begin to lose their vision should retire early.

_____ It is unsafe for an older visually impaired person to continue to use his or her stove to prepare meals.

_____ Older persons with macular degeneration will eventually become completely blind.

_____ Most older people who have one of the four leading age-related eye conditions are totally blind.

_____ Vision-related rehabilitation services are covered by Medicare and Medicaid, just as occupational and physical therapies are reimbursable by third-party insurance.

MODULE 1

The Demographics of Aging and Vision Loss: Implications for Service Delivery

This module gives an overview of the significance of the aging segment of society in the United States, its growth relative to the overall population, and its demographic characteristics with regard to vision loss. It provides definitions of key terms, data on the older population, projections to the year 2030, and an analysis of the impact of these demographics on the service delivery system for older individuals and the vision rehabilitation field in general.

Topic Outline

1.1 Demographic Data and Age-Related Vision Loss
1.2 The Growth of America's Older Population
    1.2.1 An Aging Society
    1.2.2 The Oldest Old
    1.2.3 The Aging of the Baby Boom Generation
1.3 Characteristics of the Aging Population
    1.3.1 Population Growth among Ethnic Minority Groups
    1.3.2 Marital Status and Living Arrangements
    1.3.3 Geographic Distribution
    1.3.4 Income and Poverty
    1.3.5 Employment

    1.3.6 Education

    1.3.7 Health and Health Care

1.4 Demographics of Aging and Vision: Shaping Policies and Programs

1.5 Vision-Related Statistics

    1.5.1 Data Collection

    1.5.2 Definitions of Key Terms

    1.5.3 Data Sources

    1.5.4 Estimated Prevalence and Incidence of Visual Impairment

    1.5.5 Estimated Prevalence and Incidence of Legal Blindness

    1.5.6 Estimated Rates of Visual Impairment among Older Americans

1.6 Implications of Demographic Trends

    1.6.1 Projections for the Future

    1.6.2 Impact on the Service Delivery System for Older Persons

    1.6.3 Impact on the Vision Rehabilitation Field

Learner Objectives

1. The student will be able to describe the historical growth in the aging population and the projected growth for the next three decades.
2. The student will be able to describe the increased incidence and prevalence of visual impairment among Americans age 55 and older.
3. The student will be able to describe the impact of the growth in the population of older persons experiencing age-related vision loss on service delivery systems, including the vision rehabilitation field and the aging network.

1.1 Demographic Data and Age-Related Vision Loss

Demographics are statistical measures of population characteristics. The basic set of characteristics includes age, sex, and, often, race.

These demographic features have a biological component, and they typically take on social, cultural, and even political significance. Beyond this data, there is a virtually unlimited number of biological and social characteristics about which to collect data. Degree of visual functioning is just one.

Demographics are an important part of the knowledge base about aging and age-related vision loss. The multifaceted data they provide serve as indicators of services needed now and during the early decades of the 21st century. Demographic information should inform the public policies and funding needed to develop new services and to evaluate and improve existing services.

Data collected to describe the growing and diversifying population of individuals age 65 and older in the United States typically are broken down into the following age groups: 65 and older, 75 and older, and 85 and older. Using these same age group dividers—65, 75, and 85—data are often grouped into age cohorts, which are characterized as follows: the young-old, ages 65–74; the middle-old, 75–84; and the old-old—age 85 and older.

These cohorts, first defined by Neugarten in her classic, *Middle Age and Aging* (1968), were based on common life phases characterized by typical needs. For example, people between the ages of 65 and 74 are usually newly retired and involving themselves in postretirement activities. Individuals who survive to the middle-old group, 75 to 84, characteristically are experiencing at least some health problems and limitations in physical function; and the old-old have been described as "the frail elderly" (although many individuals in this age group do not, in fact, fit this description).

Another important factor that influences the collection of data based on certain age cohorts is eligibility for services. For example, most people become eligible for Social Security and Medicare benefits at age 65. For older persons who are blind or visually impaired, it is important to collect data on individuals who are age 55 or older, because the federally funded program that provides vision rehabilitation for independent living covers individuals in that age group (see Module 4). Therefore, a fourth age cohort, ages 55 to 64, has been added to the typical set to describe the population of older persons who are blind or visually impaired (Orr, 1992).

Demographic data are central to social and medical research. Specifically, epidemiological data are concerned with how health

**MODULE 1:
THE DEMOGRAPHICS
OF AGING AND
VISION LOSS**

problems and disabling conditions are acquired. To understand the incidence of disease, for example, epidemiologists examine whether factors such as ethnicity or geographic location seem to be risk factors for certain diseases or conditions. For instance, diabetic retinopathy is associated with diabetes, which is more prevalent among the African-American and Hispanic populations.

The main focus of demographic data in this curriculum is on different age groups, degree of visual impairment and visual functioning, and, to some extent, ethnicity. Data related to income, living arrangements, health system utilization, and geographic location are also relevant because of their implications for service needs.

For example, older persons who are not eligible for Medicaid but who nevertheless have low incomes may seek medical care less frequently than would be desirable, be less likely to have access to preventive care such as routine eye examinations, and, therefore, may experience more serious vision loss than those whose eye condition is detected and treated earlier, if treatable.

To understand vision loss as it relates to the aging process, it is first important to grasp some key demographic facts related to aging. Primary characteristics that have been found to predict well-being, as well as life expectancy and problems associated with aging, include gender, ethnicity, income, source of income, marital status, living arrangements, education level, health status, hospital utilization and length of stay, and utilization of benefits and entitlement programs.

The distribution of each of these characteristics may be used to present a profile of the population; if measured at various points over time, the characteristics as measured describe trends in the population. Based on this type of statistical information, service needs can be derived, eligibility criteria established, service delivery models and methods developed, legislation enacted, and funds appropriated and allocated. The more service providers and planners know about the current and future generations of older persons, the more prepared and active they can be in meeting their needs.

The description of the aging population presented in this module is provided to establish a context for understanding the subpopulation of older people experiencing age-related vision loss. The intention is to help professionals in the fields of aging and vision rehabilitation understand the growing need to target this subpopulation and to ensure that services are available to meet its growing, changing, and diversifying needs, now and in the near future.

Solid data are an advocate's most valuable weapon. Without well-understood, reliable, and well-documented statistics, even the most compelling argument supporting the need for increased public awareness and increased resources, such as federal funding and highly trained specialized personnel, will not result in needed changes. Although anecdotal data are powerful by virtue of enabling people to understand the true nature of a problem and its profound impact, rarely do testimonials alone move decision makers to consider the next step. Hard data speak louder than anecdotal testimony—loudly enough so that funders, policymakers, and the media in influential positions are compelled to recognize the nature and extent of a problem and act accordingly.

1.2 The Growth of America's Older Population*

The United States has long been considered a nation of youth. In its colonial past, half the nation's inhabitants were under the age of 16. Most people never reached old age as we know it today. Even by 1900, life expectancy at birth was only 47 years.

Times have changed, however. Most newborns are now expected to survive their infancy, and many Americans live into their eighth decade. With improvement in health care and increased longevity come the need to reevaluate the national self-image. The United States is no longer only a nation of youth, but also one of age.

1.2.1 An Aging Society

According to the U.S. Bureau of the Census, between 1965 and 1995 the number of people age 65 or older grew by 82 percent. Between 1980 and 1996, this population grew by 28 percent to a historical high of 33.9 million people. Currently, one in eight Americans is 65 years of age or older. And, whereas less than 25 percent

---

*Unless otherwise indicated, the demographic data in this and the following section are taken from *Profile of Older Americans: 1997* (Washington, DC: American Association of Retired Persons, Program Resources Department, and Administration on Aging, U.S. Department of Health and Human Services, 1997). This information is also available on the Web site of the Administration on Aging: http://www.aoa.dhhs.gov or www.aoa.dhhs.gov/aoa/stats/profile. The term "older" refers here to people age 65 and older.

of the population is younger than age 15, another 57 percent is 30 or older (Administration on Aging, 1995). Clearly, the proportion of older citizens is growing and, with the aging of the baby boom generation as well as a recently documented lower birth rate, the United States is becoming an aging society.

Since 1900, the percentage of the U.S. population that is age 65 and older has more than tripled (from 4.1 percent in 1900 to 12.8 percent in 1996), and the number of older persons has increased nearly 11 times (from 3.1 million to 33.9 million).

The older population itself is getting older. In 1996, the 65–74 age group (18.7 million) was eight times larger than in 1900, but the 75–84 group (11.4 million) was 16 times larger, and the population aged 85 and older (3.8 million) was *31 times* larger!

In 1996, individuals reaching age 65 had an average life expectancy of an additional 17.7 years (19.2 years for females and 15.5 years for males). As a result of reduced death rates for children and young adults, the average life expectancy of a child born in 1996 is 76.1 years, almost 30 years longer than a child born in 1900.

These figures document the aging of American society, but growth in the aging population occurs not only in the United States; aging is a global phenomenon.

1.2.2 *The Oldest Old*

The "oldest-old" age group—those individuals age 85 and older—is the fastest-growing segment of America's senior citizen population. The number of persons aged 85 and older has more than doubled since 1965 and has grown by 40 percent since 1980. The number of centenarians—those 100 years and older—more than doubled during the 1980s. Although the oldest-old category currently constitutes only 1 percent of the total U.S. population, this segment is having a major impact on the nation's health care and social service delivery systems, as well as on the family unit. Many of those in the 85-and-older population have multiple health problems and other limiting physical conditions, including age-related vision loss. These individuals require the services of the health care system on an ongoing basis, including both routine visits to physicians and hospitalizations.

The family members who are most likely to care for people in this group—usually adult children—might themselves be age 60 or older. They may be beginning to experience their own health problems, may be still in the workforce, and may be caring for children still living at home. Family caregivers—adult children or even grandchildren—are less frequently living near enough to provide direct assistance themselves.

Therefore, people who are 85 and older increasingly depend on formal service delivery systems, including the aging network, home care services, and, eventually, the nursing home industry. Family caregivers must often arrange for social services and in-home assistance long distance, which creates a tremendous emotional burden.

1.2.3 The Aging of the Baby Boom Generation

Although the older population is continuing to grow, this growth slowed down to some degree during the 1990s because of the relatively small number of babies born during the Great Depression of the 1930s. That trend is expected to reverse, however, when the baby boom generation—the 75 million people born in the United States between 1946 and 1964—reaches old age.

In 1994, baby boomers represented nearly one-third the population of the United States. Between 2010 and 2030, these individuals will enter the 65-years-and-older age category. As these baby boomers begin to age, the United States will see an unparalleled increase in both the absolute number of older persons and the proportion of older persons in the overall population.

Although one in eight Americans was 65 years of age or older in 1994, by 2030 approximately one in five is expected to be age 65 or over. At that time, there will be about 70 million older persons, more than double their number in 1996. By the year 2000, people 65 and older are projected to represent 13 percent of the population, and by 2030, 20 percent. (See "A Quick Look at the U.S. Aging Population.")

In the first third of the 21st century, the older U.S. population will be characterized by experienced, educated, active, energetic people who will be less likely than previous generations to follow the "linear life" paradigm, in which people progress sequentially through the stages of education and employment, followed by retirement and leisure. This phenomenon is already being seen in American society today. People go through these stages as their interests and needs

A Quick Look at the U.S. Aging Population

- The population of persons 65 years or older numbered 33.9 million in 1996: 20.0 million older women and 13.9 million older men. They represented 12.8 percent of the U.S. population, about one in every eight Americans.
- By the year 2030, there will be about 70 million older persons, more than twice their number in 1996. The number of those age 85 and older is expected to increase from 3.8 million in 1996 to 8.5 million in 2030.
- One-quarter of the elderly population are expected to be members of minority groups in 2030, up from 13 percent in 1990.
- The median income of older persons in 1996 was $16,684 for males and $9,626 for females. After adjusting for inflation, these figures represented a decrease in real income from 1995 of 1.7 percent for men and 0.1 percent for women.
- About 3.4 million elderly persons, or 10 percent of the elderly population, lived below the poverty level in 1996. Almost one-fifth of the older population was poor or near poor.
- Older people accounted for 38 percent of all hospital stays and 48 percent of all days of care in hospitals in 1995.

Source: Profile of Older Americans: 1997 *(Washington, DC: American Association of Retired Persons, Program Resources Department, and Administration on Aging, U.S. Department of Health and Human Services, 1997). This compilation of the latest federal data on America's older population is also available on the Web page of the Administration on Aging, http://www.aoa.dhhs.gov or www.aoa.dhhs.gov/aoa/stats/profile.*

demand; many people go back to school in midlife, for example, or make midlife major career changes. According to Dychwald (1997) the United States is on the verge of becoming a "gerontocracy."

The U.S. Administration on Aging has been encouraging planners and policymakers to prepare now for the aging of the baby boomers so that the nation is poised to meet the challenges that will ensue as this unprecedentedly large generation reaches age 65. Since vision loss is a concomitant of the aging process (see Module 2), service planners and providers in the fields of aging and vision rehabilitation will have to work together to meet the increased need and demand for services that is projected.

Recently, one data source revealed that the rate of increase in the number of older persons who will be visually impaired or have other disabling conditions may not be quite as dramatic as had previously been projected (McNeil, 1997). However, in the case of age-related vision loss, the reality is that the current numbers and those projected for the next three decades are so high that it will take the service delivery systems considerable time to catch up to the need. Even with a slight decrease in the projections, the numbers of visually impaired older people will be too large to handle with the current service delivery systems.

1.3 Characteristics of the Aging Population

1.3.1 Population Growth among Ethnic Minority Groups

In 1996, approximately 15 percent of people age 65 and older were members of minority groups, inching up from 14 percent in 1994. Of these, 7.9 percent were African-American, 1.9 percent were Asian or Pacific Islander; and less than 1 percent were American Indian or Native Alaskan. Persons of Hispanic origin (who may be of any race) represented 4.7 percent of the older population. By 2030, however, persons who are members of ethnic minority groups are expected to constitute 25 percent of the elderly population.

Since members of several ethnic minority groups (African-American, Hispanic, and American Indian) experience higher rates of age-related vision loss than the population at large (National Advisory Eye Council, 1993), the projected growth in these populations will contribute to increases in the number and proportion of older people experiencing age-related vision loss. Bilingual and bicultural outreach strategies will be even more necessary than they already are to ensure that these older people have equal access to services (see Module 5).

1.3.2 Marital Status and Living Arrangements

Since the life expectancy for women is longer than that for men, the phenomenon of older women living alone has been recognized for many decades, with considerable implications for service delivery. Older women in their last decade of life are less likely to have the in-home support and assistance of a spouse, and are more likely to depend on adult children, friends and neighbors, or formal service delivery systems for help.

In 1996, there were 20 million older women (age 65 and older) and 13.9 million older men, or a ratio of 145 women for every 100 men. The ratio of women to men increases with age.

In 1995, older men were much more likely to be married than older women—76 percent of men, 43 percent of women. Almost half of all older women in 1995 were widows, and there were five times as many widows as widowers. Divorced older persons represented only 6 percent of all older persons in 1995, but the number of divorced older persons had increased three times as fast as the older population as a whole since 1990.

The majority of older persons who were not living in institutions (67 percent) lived with family members in 1995 (approximately 81 percent of older men and 57 percent of older women); however, the proportion living in a family setting decreased with age, primarily due to the death of a spouse. An additional 2 percent lived with people who were not relatives, and about 30 percent of all noninstitutionalized older persons lived alone (42 percent of older women and 17 percent of older men).

Although only a small number of those age 65 and older lived in nursing homes (1.4 million or 4 percent), the percentage increased dramatically with age, ranging from 1 percent for persons aged 65–74 years to 5 percent for persons 75–84 years and 15 percent for persons 85 and older. The most significant predictor of nursing home placement is the lack of informal caregivers that would make it possible to remain at home.

1.3.3 Geographic Distribution

In 1996, about half of all persons age 65 and older lived in 9 states. California had over 3 million, Florida and New York had over 2 million each, and Texas, Pennsylvania, Ohio, Illinois, Michigan, and New Jersey each had over 1 million. The growing proportion of older residents has challenged these states in particular and their aging service networks to be more comprehensive in the provision of services and the development of structures for service delivery.

1.3.4 Income and Poverty

Of all older persons reporting annual income in 1996 (31.2 million), 40 percent reported less than $10,000, and the median income reported was $12,214. Only 18 percent reported income of $25,000 or more. The major sources of income were Social Security retirement income (reported by 92 percent of older persons), income from property or assets (reported by 66 percent), public and private pensions (reported by 32 percent), earnings (reported by 16 percent), and public assistance (reported by 5 percent).

About 3.4 million elderly persons were below the federally defined poverty level in 1996. The poverty rate for persons age 65 and older was 10.8 percent, slightly less than the rate for persons aged 18–64 (11.4 percent). Another 2.4 million or 7.6 percent of the elderly were classified as "near-poor" (income between the poverty level and 125 percent of this level). In total, almost one-fifth (18.4 percent) of the older population was poor or near-poor in 1996.

Older women had a higher poverty rate (13.6 percent) than older men (6.8 percent), and older persons living alone or with nonrelatives were more likely to be poor (20.8 percent) than were older persons living with families (6.0 percent).

One of every 11 (9.4 percent) elderly white individuals was poor in 1996, compared to one-fourth (25.3 percent) of elderly African-Americans and almost one-fourth (24.4 percent) of elderly Hispanics. Almost one-half (47.5 percent) of older black women who lived alone were poor.

Income is an important predictor of access to services and an older person's ability to take advantage of existing services, particularly health services and preventive care. Thus, those who are least well-off financially are more likely to have multiple and complex health problems because they are less able to purchase care. There is a close correlation between being an older woman who lives alone or is a member of an ethnic minority group and low income.

1.3.5 Employment

About 3.8 million older Americans (12 percent) were in the labor force in 1997—defined as employed or actively seeking employment—including 17 percent of the men and 8 percent of the women. They constituted 2.7 percent of the U.S. labor force. About 3.4 percent of them were unemployed.

The limited number of employment opportunities for older persons in general has a significant impact on the number of older people who are visually impaired who want to remain in or reenter the workforce. Since work opportunities are limited, it is more difficult for the newly visually impaired older person to receive vocational rehabilitation than it is to obtain rehabilitation services for independent living training (see Module 3). Even though an older individual may express a work-oriented goal when applying for services, he or she will have more difficulty in justifying the validity of the goal than will someone of traditional working age.

It is also important to note that even within the population of individuals of typical working age who are blind or visually impaired, approximately 70 percent are unemployed (McNeil, 1997), despite a slight recent trend toward higher rates of employment. The unemployed include individuals who are encouraged to take early retirement or who choose it themselves because they are unaware of the range of vision-related rehabilitation services and adaptive technology available to enable newly visually impaired people to remain in the workforce (see Module 6).

1.3.6 Education

The educational level of the older population is increasing. Between 1970 and 1995, the percentage who had completed high school rose from 28 percent to 64 percent. About 13 percent had at least a bachelor's degree. The percentage who had completed high school varied considerably by race and ethnic origin: 67 percent of whites, 37 percent of African-Americans, and 30 percent of the Hispanic population.

Thus, the older Americans of the 21st century will have higher educational levels, and, consequently, increased access to information, greater exposure to and knowledge of technology, expanded awareness of available services, and improved skills in obtaining information and services. In other words, the next generation of older people is likely to make greater demands for services, including vision-related services and adaptive technology. Service providers and those in decision-making positions need to plan now for a more assertive cohort of older persons with stronger self-advocacy skills.

1.3.7 Health and Health Care

In 1994, 28 percent of older persons assessed their health as fair or poor, compared to 10 percent for all persons. There was little difference between the sexes on this measure, but older African-Americans were much more likely to rate their health as fair or poor (43 percent) than were older whites (27 percent).

In 1992, more than half of the older population (53.9 percent) reported having at least one disability that limited them in carrying out activities of daily living and instrumental activities of daily living. (Activities of daily living include bathing, toileting, transferring from bed to a chair, dressing, eating, and getting around the house. Instrumental activities of daily living include preparing meals, shopping, managing money, using the telephone, and doing housework.) Over 5 million older people need assistance with activities of daily living, and the percentage needing help increases sharply with age.

Most older persons have at least one chronic health condition and many have multiple conditions. The most frequently occurring conditions in 1994 were arthritis (occurring in 50 percent of noninstitutionalized elderly people), hypertension (in 36 percent), heart disease (in 32 percent), hearing impairments (in 29 percent), cataracts (in 17 percent), orthopedic impairments (in 16 percent), sinusitis (in 15 percent), and diabetes (in 10 percent).

Approximately two-thirds of older people who experience age-related vision loss have at least one other condition that limits their independent mobility and their ability to carry out various instrumental activities of daily living. The effects of vision loss either compound or are compounded by the other disabling conditions.

1.4 Demographics of Aging and Vision: Shaping Policies and Programs

As already noted, because vision loss frequently accompanies the aging process, the rapid growth in the population of older people in the United States has likewise resulted in a sharp rise in both the number and proportion of blind and visually impaired people who are elderly. This dramatic demographic shift in the population of people who are blind and visually impaired has created a new reality for agencies in the field of blindness and vision rehabilitation as well as for the aging network—those agencies that provide services to the general population of aging individuals.

The "graying" of the potential client population presents a challenge to the vision-related rehabilitation service delivery system to meet the needs of this group. Although this has been a concern for the last quarter of the 20th century, funding and personnel resources in the vision rehabilitation field have traditionally been directed more toward education and employment than to the needs of older persons. However, services and methods of service delivery that target rehabilitation related to vocational goals can no longer meet the changing and diversifying needs of older people who are experiencing age-related vision loss.

Agencies in the field of vision-related rehabilitation also face the challenge of working in cooperation with the aging network, the health care system, and related fields. All disciplines that serve this population need to collaborate in examining and redesigning services and service delivery methods to meet their growing numbers. Mutual understanding among professionals across many disciplines and services along a continuum of care are needed to serve this population.

1.5 Vision-Related Statistics

1.5.1 Data Collection

As a basis for providing services to older people who are visually impaired, it is first necessary to know the size and composition of this population. And, although this curriculum focuses on older adults, age 55 and over, it is important to also look at data on the overall U.S. population that is experiencing some degree of visual impairment to obtain a broad picture of the subpopulation and how the demographics change as individuals age.

Yet, when dealing with blindness and visual impairment, these are not easy questions to answer, for several reasons. First, visual impairment is difficult to define precisely. Whereas total blindness is easier to conceptualize, what a visually impaired individual can and cannot see may vary from day to day and is influenced by the environmental circumstances and the kind of eyeglasses or other optical devices used. Furthermore, two people with the same clinical measure of visual acuity may have different visual abilities—and the same individual may see differently depending on fatigue or the time of day. Yet because today the vast majority of individuals with vision problems have some usable vision under certain circumstances, it is important to describe and define visual impairment so that it can be understood by the general public and professionals alike.

Second, it has been difficult to collect accurate data on the numbers of older people with varying degrees of vision loss. The accuracy of attempts to collect this information during census taking and national surveys about health status has been affected by the threatening and potentially stigmatizing nature of the condition (see Module 3). It is difficult for an individual to identify with and acknowledge blindness and even more difficult to admit it to others. Thus, an older person is not likely to respond affirmatively to a direct question such as, "Are you or any member of your household blind?"

Questions that are based on functional ability such as, "Do you or any member of your household have any difficulty reading newspaper print?" are considerably less threatening and are likely to result in more accurate responses (see the discussion of definitions of terms in the next section). However, different surveys have used different definitions, making it necessary to understand the meaning behind the categories in order to be able to compare data sets.

Because collecting precise data on visual impairment is so crucial in determining the real need for services, the American Foundation for the Blind (AFB) has been working with the methods laboratories of the two federal agencies that conduct relevant surveys large enough to yield helpful estimates—the U.S. Bureau of the Census and the National Center for Health Statistics (NCHS)—to improve and make consistent one of the key measures of visual impairment of use to the field.

Despite improvement in data collection over the last few decades through more accurate sampling and phrasing of questions related to vision problems, it is also important to note that many statistics reflect a serious undercount of the numbers of older people who are blind or visually impaired.

1.5.2 Definitions of Key Terms

In general, data on visual impairment are reported as either prevalence data or incidence data.

- *Prevalence* refers to the number of individuals who fall into a given category at a given point in time, usually a year; for example, the number of individuals in 1998 age 55 and older who have a visual acuity of 20/200 or less.
- *Incidence* refers to the number of *new* cases of vision loss during a given time period, usually a year, such as the number of individuals age 55 and older with visual acuity of 20/200 or less who acquired that status during 1997.

- *Rates* for prevalence and incidence are determined by the prevalence number or the incidence number divided by the total population in a given category (the total U.S. population unless stated otherwise). Rates are usually expressed as percentages (the number of individuals per hundred) or as the number of individuals per thousand.

The definitions used for the statistics presented here may seem complex. However, they are chosen to keep the wording close to the terminology and definitions actually used in studies—for example, by the Bureau of the Census—so that the results can be easily linked to the source of the data.

Vision loss can be described in two primary ways. It is frequently defined by *clinical* measures such as visual acuity (see Module 2), using tools such as the familiar eye chart. However, a *functional* definition that is based on how visual impairment affects the individual's day-to-day activities is more easily understood by the general public. It is also more relevant to determining the need for rehabilitation services, which are intended to improve functioning.

For example, degree of vision loss may be described or defined with regard to reading print as "has difficulty reading printed material" or "is unable to read print." These terms convey the impact of vision loss on an individual's ability to function—to carry out activities of daily living and instrumental activities of daily living. They give information about an individual that others can easily comprehend and that helps the user of the data think about the kind of help the individual may require.

Although the number of activities that might be used to measure functional vision is almost endless, in contemporary society reading print is a basic function. In addition, vision problems that make it difficult to read print can also indicate the degree of difficulty one might have in a wide range of other activities.

Thus, the major surveys that attempt to measure functional vision loss focus on reading and attempt to standardize the question by referring to the print size typically used in newspapers. However, the surveys differ somewhat in the specific wording they use and the context in which the questions appear—for example, whether the survey focuses on health issues or on economic issues. Different definitions can yield different data, since people are sometimes classified into one category or another based on subtle nuances.

In the statistics presented in this module, functional vision loss is measured at two levels: *nonsevere functional limitation* and *severe functional limitation.*

- *Severe functional limitation* refers to people who said they are *unable* to see words and letters in ordinary print, even when wearing their eyeglasses or contact lenses.
- *Nonsevere functional limitation* refers to people who report having *difficulty* seeing words and letters in ordinary print, even when wearing their eyeglasses or contact lenses.

The two categories are not mutually exclusive; the number who had *difficulty* seeing includes those who were *unable* to see words and letters.

1.5.3 Data Sources

One source of data on the prevalence of visual impairment is the U.S. Bureau of the Census. The Census Bureau conducts a periodic survey known as the Survey of Income and Program Participation (SIPP) (McNeil, 1993). This survey measures visual impairment through self-reports or proxy reports of severe and nonsevere "limitations in seeing words and letters"—that is, "print disability" that is not corrected by ordinary eyeglasses. (The survey excludes people in nursing homes and other institutional settings. Questions about seeing print were not asked for children under the age of 15 until 1994–95.) A rationale for taking estimates of the prevalence of visual impairment from SIPP data is that these figures can then be related to statistics collected in the same survey on other characteristics that are important for policy, notably employment, earnings, poverty status, and the like.

Another primary data source is the National Center for Health Statistics (NCHS), which conducts the annual Health Interview Survey (HIS). HIS data on visual impairment are especially useful for purposes related to health status, but HIS uses somewhat different definitions of severe and nonsevere visual impairment (inability to see to read ordinary newspaper print even with eyeglasses or contact lenses).*

---

*Because HIS measures severe print disability only rarely, researchers at AFB calculated the 1990 estimates presented here using formulas based on data from earlier years (see Nelson & Dimitrova, 1993).

1.5.4 Estimated Prevalence and Incidence of Visual Impairment

The figures presented here are various estimates of the prevalence and incidence of functional visual impairment in the United States during the early 1990s. Apparent discrepancies in the figures from the same source result from rounding at different stages of data analysis.

1. Estimated total adults (ages 16 and older) with severe functional limitation in seeing print (based on SIPP data), 1991–92 (McNeil, 1993):
   Number: 1.6 million
   Rate: 0.6 percent, or 6 individuals per 1,000

2. Estimated persons (all ages) with severe visual impairment (based on HIS data), 1990 (Nelson & Dimitrova, 1993):
   Number: 4.3 million
   Rate: 2 percent, or 17 per 1,000

3. Estimated total adults with functional limitation in seeing print, including both severe and nonsevere functional limitations, 1991–92 (McNeil, 1993):
   Number: 9.7 million
   Rate: 4 percent or 40 per 1,000

4. Estimated persons (all ages) with severe and nonsevere visual impairment (based on HIS data), 1990 ("Current Estimates from the National Health Interview Survey, 1990," 1991):
   Number: 7.5 million
   Rate: 4 percent, or 40 per 1,000

5. Persons of traditional working age (ages 21–64) who are severely visually impaired (based on SIPP data), 1991–92 (McNeil, 1993):
   Number: 560,000
   Rate: about 1/3 of the severely visually impaired population

6. People aged 65 or older with severe functional limitation in seeing (based on 1993–94 SIPP data) (J. M. McNeil, personal communication, February 1997):
   Number: 1.0 million
   Rate: 3 percent, or 30 per 1,000
               about 2/3 of the severely visually impaired population

7. Estimated incidence (new cases) of persons with severe functional limitation in seeing (based on SIPP data), 1991–92 (McNeil, 1993) (incidence is assumed to be about 10 percent of prevalence):
   Number: 200,000
   Rate: about 1 per 1,000

Blindness, including severe visual impairment, has been classified as a low incidence disability in comparison to other types of disabilities. As a result, it has received neither the attention nor the funding that some other conditions have attracted. However, since increasing numbers of older people experience varying degrees of vision loss as they reach their seventies and eighties, this is no longer the case. The data document the need to assign a higher priority to funding and services for older people who are blind or visually impaired.

1.5.5 Estimated Prevalence and Incidence of Legal Blindness

Legal blindness is defined clinically as a visual acuity of 20/200 or less in the better eye with the best possible correction, or a visual field of no more than 20 degrees. An individual whose vision is 20/200 sees at 20 feet what an individual with 20/20 vision can see at 200 feet. (See Module 2 and the Glossary for a detailed explanation of these terms.)

The classification of legal blindness helps to determine eligibility for some vision rehabilitation services.

People who are classified as legally blind represent a broad range of visual acuities and functional abilities or limitations, from total blindness to light perception only to 20/200 vision. Most legally blind people have some useful vision.

1. Estimated legally blind persons (all ages), c. 1990 (Chiang, Bassi, & Javitt, 1992):
   Number: 1.1 million
   Rate: 4.5 per 1,000

2. Estimated legally blind persons with some useful vision, c. 1990 (Kirchner, 1996):
   Number: 880,000
   Rate: 80 percent of legally blind persons
                  3.6 per 1,000

3. Estimated legally blind persons with no useful vision (light perception or less), c. 1990 (Kirchner, 1996):

Number: 220,000
Rate: 20 percent of legally blind persons
0.9 per 1,000

4. Estimated legally blind persons who are totally blind (no light perception), c. 1990 (Kirchner, 1996):
Number: 110,000
Rate: 10 percent of legally blind persons
0.45 per 1,000

5. Estimated incidence (new cases) of legal blindness, c. 1990 (Kirchner, 1996):
Number: 80,000
Rate: 3.3 per 10,000

1.5.6 Estimated Rates of Visual Impairment among Older Americans

Table 1 presents data about visual impairment among older people in the United States, broken down by age group. The table is based on data from the Bureau of the Census, using the SIPP definitions of severe and nonsevere functional limitation in seeing described earlier in this module.

In reading the table, it is important to note that the age categories overlap. For example, the number of people who are 55 and older also includes all those who are 65 and older, 75 and older, and 85 and older.

Table 1.1
Prevalence of Visual Impairment in Older Persons in the United States, 1995

Age Range	U.S. Population (1995)	Nonsevere Visual Impairment (including severe) Number	Rate	Severe Visual Impairment (including blindness) Number	Rate
55 & older	54,666,000	6,493,490	12%	1,230,370	2%
65 & older	33,537,000	5,087,450	15%	1,026,030	3%
75 & older	14,777,000	3,377,560	23%	749,010	5%
85 & older	3,628,000	1,277,900	35%	339,590	9%

Source: American Foundation for the Blind, Department of Policy Research and Program Evaluation, New York, 1997, based on data from U.S. Bureau of the Census, *Model-Based Estimates of Specific Disabilities for States and Counties*, www.census.gov/hhes/www/disable.html (1997); and unpublished data from the 1993–94 Survey of Income and Program Participation, John M. McNeil, personal communication, February 1997.

Similarly, because of the way the SIPP questions are phrased, the estimate for nonsevere functional limitation in seeing includes the severe functional limitation. Estimates for nonoverlapping categories (for example, for those aged 55–64 only or for those with nonsevere visual impairment only) can be calculated from the figures in the table by subtraction.

A state-by-state breakdown of these data can be found in the appendix to this module. State data are extremely important to the field of vision rehabilitation and the aging network in planning services for each state's older population. State data serve as a critical resource in advocating for adequate levels of federal and state funding for vision-related rehabilitation services for a given state. These data are also important for the aging network in planning home- and community-based long-term services within the state planning area (see Module 5).

As the figures in Table 1 indicate, even among older individuals, the prevalence of vision loss increases sharply with increasing age. The four age cohorts themselves constitute extremely diverse populations in regard to their needs, wants, and interests.

1.6 Implications of Demographic Trends

1.6.1 Projections for the Future

The demographics of aging and vision loss within the United States and the phenomenon of "global aging" are slowly beginning to shape both public policy and service delivery for this population. However, much remains to be done.

As already noted, projections indicate that by the year 2030, there will be approximately double the number of severely visually impaired persons age 65 years or older as there have been in the 1990s. The dramatic increase in this population makes it impossible to overlook the growing number of older persons who are already experiencing vision loss but are not receiving the services they require. This population requires the attention of policymakers, funders, service providers, and planners now and to plan for the decades to come.

Since the 1970s, when the growth in the aging population became very apparent, projections have been made about the number of older people who would be visually impaired by the year

2000. It is interesting to note that in each decade the actual figures have surpassed the predictions.

Both the unprecedented growth and the diversity of the elderly visually impaired population requires that agencies not only make their needs a priority but also serve them creatively and comprehensively.

Effective service delivery depends on the following critical elements:

- consumer involvement in all phases of planning and delivering of services
- an understanding that older people with impaired vision are consumers of both the aging network and the vision rehabilitation field
- collaboration among service providers to ensure comprehensive and holistic rehabilitation and supportive services
- collaborative planning and service delivery to maximize scarce resources on behalf of consumers

These themes are discussed in more detail in Modules 2 through 7.

1.6.2 Impact on the Service Delivery System for Older Persons

Because of the growing number of older people experiencing varying degrees of vision loss, service providers in the aging arena are increasingly encountering these individuals at their agencies and programs. The growth in this population has serious implications for the range of home- and community-based long-term services available to older persons and individuals with disabilities.

Often, older individuals with impaired vision seek advice from a professional at an agency serving the elderly. Service providers need to understand how to serve this group effectively within the aging network; they also must become familiar with the vision-related services available, understand the vision rehabilitation system and its eligibility criteria, and be able to make effective referrals on behalf of these older individuals who are consumers of both service delivery systems.

1.6.3 Impact on the Vision Rehabilitation Field

Each year, only a fraction of the newly visually impaired older population seeks and receives vision rehabilitation services. Five to seven years may pass from the onset of vision loss before older people seek services.

In 1995, only about 22,000 older individuals with visual impairments received vision-related rehabilitation services funded by Title VII, Chapter 2 of the Rehabilitation Act, the Independent Living Services for Older Individuals Who Are Blind program (Stephens, 1996), because of the program's limited funding level (see Module 4). This number is meager in comparison to the millions of older Americans who experience age-related vision loss and are eligible for services.

Thus, an emphasis on strategic outreach is needed for two general purposes. One is to publicize vision rehabilitation services available for older people within the community in order to increase referrals for service. The other is to contact hard-to-reach special populations, particularly the growing numbers of older people who are members of minority groups or living in rural areas who have less access to services because of language, cultural, or geographic barriers to services.

Blindness and visual impairment touch the lives of 44 million Americans when friends, colleagues, and family members—spouses and adult children in particular—are counted (*Lighthouse National Survey on Vision Loss*, 1995). All of these people benefit from specialized vision-related rehabilitation services and from the level of independence and self-reliance achieved by the older individuals who receive them.

Specialized rehabilitation services enable older persons with visual impairments to maintain full and productive lives and to maximize their ability to live independently. Vision-related rehabilitation services, discussed in greater detail in Module 4, provide older people who are blind or visually impaired with the skills they need to function as independently and productively as possible for as long as possible.

References

Administration on Aging. (1995). *The aging population.* Washington, DC: U.S. Department of Health and Human Services.

Chiang, Y., Bassi, L. J., & Javitt, J. C. (1992). Federal budgetary costs of blindness. *Milbank Quarterly, 70*(2), 319–340.

Current estimates from the National Health Interview Survey, 1990. (1991). *Vital and Health Statistics,* Series 10. Hyattsville, MD: Centers for Disease Control and Prevention, National Center for Health Statistics.

Dychwald, K. (1997). Gerontocracy, Gerassic Park and other possible consequences of an aging society. *Innovations in Aging, 26*(2), 16–18.

Kirchner, C. (1989). Unpublished memorandum. New York: American Foundation for the Blind, Social Research Group.

Kirchner, C. (1996). Unpublished memorandum. New York: American Foundation for the Blind, Department of Policy Research and Program Evaluation.

Lighthouse national survey on vision loss: The experience, attitudes and knowledge of middle-aged and older Americans. (1995). New York: The Lighthouse.

McNeil, J. M. (1993). Americans with disabilities: 1991–92: Data from the Survey of Income and Program Participation. *Current Population Reports, Household Economic Studies* (P70–33). Washington, DC: U.S. Bureau of the Census.

McNeil, J. M. (1997). Americans with disabilities: 1994–95. *Current Population Reports, Household Economic Studies* (P70-61). Washington: DC: U.S. Bureau of the Census.

National Advisory Eye Council. (1993). *Vision research: A national plan, 1994–1998.* Bethesda, MD: National Eye Institute, National Institutes of Health.

Nelson, K. A., & Dimitrova, G. (1993). Severe visual impairment in the United States and in each state, 1990. *Journal of Visual Impairment & Blindness, 87*(3), 80–85.

Neugarten, B. (Ed.). (1968). *Middle age and aging: Reader in social psychology.* Chicago: University of Chicago Press.

Orr, A. L. (1992). Aging and blindness: Toward a systems approach to service delivery. In A. L. Orr (Ed.), *Vision and aging: Crossroads for service delivery* (pp. 3–31). New York: American Foundation for the Blind.

Profile of older Americans: 1997. (1997). Washington, DC: American Association of Retired Persons, Program Resources Department and Administration on Aging, U.S. Department of Health and Human Services.

Stephens, B. (1996). *Independent living services for older individuals who are blind: Annual report for FY 1995.* Mississippi State: Mississippi State University, Rehabilitation Research and Training Center on Blindness and Low Vision.

RECOMMENDED TEACHING METHODS

Guest Speakers

Invite guest speakers from public and private agencies for blind and visually impaired persons to provide students with a description of how the public agencies (state rehabilitation agency and its local offices) use state data to plan service delivery for now and the future.

If available, invite professionals from the community who have developed an innovative or state-of-the-art service delivery package designed to meet the growing and diversifying population of older persons who are blind or visually impaired.

Small-Group Activity

Have students work in small groups to find out the statistics for their state in some of the categories of demographic data presented in this module. Have them identify the components of a service plan that would meet the specific needs of the state's population of older persons who are visually impaired.

True/False Quiz

Administer the true/false pretest about blindness and visual impairment that appears in the Introduction.

Field Trip: Agency Visit

As time and resources permit, have students visit a rehabilitation agency to understand firsthand the nature of service delivery. This can be scheduled in addition to or instead of having guest lectures in the classroom. One recommended approach is to invite a guest from the state rehabilitation agency and have students visit a private agency that serves people who are blind or visually impaired.

MODULE 1:
THE DEMOGRAPHICS
OF AGING AND
VISION LOSS

APPENDIX

Estimated Rates of Visual Impairment among Older Americans

The Census Bureau publishes estimates of the number of persons with various functional limitations by state and county. These estimates, along with a description of the methodology, are available on the World Wide Web at www.census.gov. However, the census estimates do not present state data by age. In order to provide state data by age, age-specific national estimates were obtained from the Census Bureau. The state estimates were combined with the age-specific national estimates to calculate the figures for the tables.

Estimated Rates of Visual Impairment among Older Americans by State, 1995

State	Age Range	State Population (1995)	Nonsevere Visual Impairment (including severe) Number	Rate	Severe Visual Impairment (including blindness) Number	Rate
AK	55 & older	68,000	4,590	7%	720	1%
	65 & older	30,000	2,830	9%	490	2%
	75 & older	10,000	1,550	16%	300	3%
	85 & older	2,000	500	25%	120	6%
AL	55 & older	927,000	147,530	16%	31,630	3%
	65 & older	552,000	113,650	21%	26,050	5%
	75 & older	240,000	74,920	31%	18,910	8%
	85 & older	58,000	28,030	48%	8,490	15%
AR	55 & older	583,000	93,960	16%	19,780	3%
	65 & older	360,000	74,240	21%	16,630	5%
	75 & older	164,000	50,420	31%	12,380	8%
	85 & older	41,000	19,400	47%	5,700	14%
AZ	55 & older	886,000	85,740	10%	15,120	2%
	65 & older	560,000	67,970	12%	12,710	2%
	75 & older	237,000	43,780	18%	9,020	4%
	85 & older	51,000	14,870	29%	3,720	7%
CA	55 & older	5,647,000	591,870	10%	105,190	2%
	65 & older	3,463,000	463,250	13%	87,650	3%
	75 & older	1,496,000	304,060	20%	63,400	4%
	85 & older	359,000	113,110	32%	28,340	8%
CO	55 & older	673,000	58,790	9%	10,280	2%

APPENDIX: ESTIMATED RATES OF VISUAL IMPAIRMENT AMONG OLDER AMERICANS

State	Age Range	State Population (1995)	Nonsevere Visual Impairment (including severe) Number	Rate	Severe Visual Impairment (including blindness) Number	Rate
	65 & older	375,000	43,530	12%	8,210	2%
	75 & older	159,000	28,330	18%	5,910	4%
	85 & older	40,000	10,960	27%	2,730	7%
CT	55 & older	734,000	73,420	10%	13,130	2%
	65 & older	467,000	59,050	13%	11,190	2%
	75 & older	217,000	40,560	19%	8,400	4%
	85 & older	54,000	15,550	29%	3,860	7%
DC	55 & older	122,000	22,140	18%	4,320	4%
	65 & older	77,000	17,680	23%	3,660	5%
	75 & older	34,000	11,830	35%	2,700	8%
	85 & older	9,000	4,770	53%	1,290	14%
DE	55 & older	149,000	18,770	13%	3,450	2%
	65 & older	91,000	14,590	16%	2,860	3%
	75 & older	37,000	9,230	25%	2,010	5%
	85 & older	9,000	3,470	39%	910	10%
FL	55 & older	3,886,000	543,200	14%	100,790	3%
	65 & older	2,631,000	449,550	17%	87,640	3%
	75 & older	1,172,000	299,930	26%	64,170	5%
	85 & older	271,000	108,190	40%	27,910	10%
GA	55 & older	1,259,000	177,690	14%	36,320	3%
	65 & older	718,000	133,180	19%	29,260	4%
	75 & older	306,000	86,600	28%	20,990	7%
	85 & older	72,000	31,690	44%	9,250	13%
HI	55 & older	243,000	20,710	9%	3,630	1%
	65 & older	150,000	16,130	11%	3,010	2%
	75 & older	60,000	10,030	17%	2,080	3%
	85 & older	13,000	3,430	26%	860	7%
IA	55 & older	680,000	70,860	10%	12,620	2%
	65 & older	432,000	57,350	13%	10,830	3%
	75 & older	211,000	40,810	19%	8,390	4%
	85 & older	59,000	17,200	29%	4,180	7%
ID	55 & older	225,000	20,990	9%	3,670	2%
	65 & older	132,000	16,080	12%	3,010	2%
	75 & older	60,000	10,870	18%	2,230	4%
	85 & older	14,000	3,950	28%	970	7%
IL	55 & older	2,436,000	261,520	11%	48,620	2%
	65 & older	1,484,000	204,940	14%	40,610	3%
	75 & older	671,000	138,530	21%	30,110	4%
	85 & older	167,000	53,100	32%	13,820	8%

(continued on following page)

Estimated Rates of Visual Impairment *(continued)*

State	Age Range	State Population (1995)	Nonsevere Visual Impairment (including severe) Number	Rate	Severe Visual Impairment (including blindness) Number	Rate
IN	55 & older	1,220,000	125,190	10%	23,120	2%
	65 & older	734,000	97,210	13%	19,160	3%
	75 & older	323,000	64,690	20%	14,030	4%
	85 & older	81,000	24,950	31%	6,470	8%
KS	55 & older	553,000	57,580	10%	10,360	2%
	65 & older	350,000	46,430	13%	8,870	3%
	75 & older	167,000	32,610	20%	6,800	4%
	85 & older	47,000	13,810	29%	3,400	7%
KY	55 & older	825,000	128,510	16%	27,500	3%
	65 & older	487,000	98,560	20%	22,570	5%
	75 & older	212,000	65,080	31%	16,410	8%
	85 & older	52,000	24,650	47%	7,450	14%
LA	55 & older	845,000	137,640	16%	28,350	3%
	65 & older	494,000	104,640	21%	23,080	5%
	75 & older	209,000	67,800	32%	16,520	8%
	85 & older	50,000	25,160	50%	7,370	15%
MA	55 & older	1,332,000	139,180	10%	25,960	2%
	65 & older	861,000	113,010	13%	22,300	3%
	75 & older	400,000	77,810	19%	16,790	4%
	85 & older	104,000	30,910	30%	7,950	8%
MD	55 & older	963,000	123,530	13%	23,130	2%
	65 & older	572,000	94,680	17%	18,950	3%
	75 & older	240,000	61,010	25%	13,500	6%
	85 & older	57,000	22,500	39%	5,990	11%
ME	55 & older	277,000	29,530	11%	5,480	2%
	65 & older	174,000	23,560	14%	4,650	3%
	75 & older	78,000	15,920	20%	3,450	4%
	85 & older	21,000	6,510	31%	1,680	8%
MI	55 & older	1,945,000	212,340	11%	39,880	2%
	65 & older	1,182,000	165,360	14%	33,100	3%
	75 & older	512,000	108,670	21%	23,960	5%
	85 & older	122,000	40,190	33%	10,650	9%
MN	55 & older	925,000	91,070	10%	16,040	2%
	65 & older	572,000	72,550	13%	13,600	2%
	75 & older	275,000	51,130	19%	10,450	4%
	85 & older	76,000	21,340	28%	5,160	7%
MO	55 & older	1,192,000	133,120	11%	25,570	2%
	65 & older	740,000	105,800	14%	21,620	3%

APPENDIX: ESTIMATED RATES OF VISUAL IMPAIRMENT AMONG OLDER AMERICANS

State	Age Range	State Population (1995)	Nonsevere Visual Impairment (including severe) Number	Rate	Severe Visual Impairment (including blindness) Number	Rate
	75 & older	341,000	72,660	21%	16,270	5%
	85 & older	92,000	29,750	32%	7,910	9%
MS	55 & older	553,000	98,340	18%	21,630	4%
	65 & older	331,000	76,210	23%	17,910	5%
	75 & older	147,000	51,000	35%	13,180	9%
	85 & older	37,000	19,730	53%	6,100	16%
MT	55 & older	191,000	18,370	10%	3,200	2%
	65 & older	114,000	14,260	13%	2,660	2%
	75 & older	53,000	9,790	18%	1,990	4%
	85 & older	13,000	3,710	29%	910	7%
NC	55 & older	1,508,000	211,820	14%	42,880	3%
	65 & older	899,000	162,540	18%	35,150	4%
	75 & older	376,000	104,370	28%	24,950	7%
	85 & older	87,000	37,670	43%	10,860	12%
ND	55 & older	146,000	15,010	10%	2,530	2%
	65 & older	93,000	12,200	13%	2,180	2%
	75 & older	47,000	8,840	19%	1,710	4%
	85 & older	13,000	3,690	28%	850	7%
NE	55 & older	362,000	36,950	10%	6,370	2%
	65 & older	228,000	29,770	13%	5,450	2%
	75 & older	110,000	21,080	19%	4,210	4%
	85 & older	32,000	9,170	29%	2,160	7%
NH	55 & older	219,000	20,650	9%	3,670	2%
	65 & older	136,000	16,320	12%	3,080	2%
	75 & older	60,000	10,880	18%	2,260	4%
	85 & older	15,000	4,190	28%	1,040	7%
NJ	55 & older	1,761,000	179,960	10%	32,790	2%
	65 & older	1,091,000	141,810	13%	27,470	3%
	75 & older	478,000	93,840	20%	20,000	4%
	85 & older	114,000	34,730	30%	8,900	8%
NM	55 & older	318,000	34,370	11%	6,040	2%
	65 & older	183,000	25,840	14%	4,880	3%
	75 & older	76,000	16,540	22%	3,460	5%
	85 & older	18,000	6,090	34%	1,530	8%
NV	55 & older	309,000	24,070	8%	4,110	1%
	65 & older	176,000	17,660	10%	3,230	2%
	75 & older	64,000	10,240	16%	2,100	3%
	85 & older	12,000	3,090	26%	780	6%
NY	55 & older	3,958,000	452,420	11%	84,870	2%

(continued on following page)

MODULE 1:
THE DEMOGRAPHICS
OF AGING AND
VISION LOSS

Estimated Rates of Visual Impairment *(continued)*

State	Age Range	State Population (1995)	Nonsevere Visual Impairment (including severe) Number	Rate	Severe Visual Impairment (including blindness) Number	Rate
	65 & older	2,424,000	355,300	15%	71,010	3%
	75 & older	1,075,000	237,920	22%	52,300	5%
	85 & older	277,000	93,830	34%	24,600	9%
OH	55 & older	2,435,000	261,750	11%	49,090	2%
	65 & older	1,491,000	204,870	14%	40,920	3%
	75 & older	649,000	135,150	21%	29,720	5%
	85 & older	157,000	50,610	32%	13,360	9%
OK	55 & older	732,000	107,680	15%	21,590	3%
	65 & older	443,000	84,240	19%	18,020	4%
	75 & older	201,000	57,250	28%	13,440	7%
	85 & older	53,000	23,010	43%	6,430	12%
OR	55 & older	681,000	67,060	10%	12,120	2%
	65 & older	426,000	53,350	13%	10,240	2%
	75 & older	196,000	36,360	19%	7,630	4%
	85 & older	47,000	13,520	29%	3,410	7%
PA	55 & older	2,969,000	324,720	11%	60,860	2%
	65 & older	1,916,000	261,950	14%	51,920	3%
	75 & older	852,000	174,780	21%	38,040	4%
	85 & older	201,000	64,110	32%	16,790	8%
RI	55 & older	231,000	25,770	11%	4,780	2%
	65 & older	156,000	21,380	14%	4,170	3%
	75 & older	72,000	14,630	20%	3,120	4%
	85 & older	18,000	5,630	31%	1,440	8%
SC	55 & older	745,000	109,380	15%	22,190	3%
	65 & older	440,000	83,190	19%	18,050	4%
	75 & older	179,000	52,400	29%	12,600	7%
	85 & older	40,000	18,370	46%	5,340	13%
SD	55 & older	164,000	17,020	10%	2,920	2%
	65 & older	105,000	13,820	13%	2,510	2%
	75 & older	51,000	9,790	19%	1,940	4%
	85 & older	14,000	4,060	29%	950	7%
TN	55 & older	1,120,000	165,920	15%	34,600	3%
	65 & older	658,000	126,860	19%	28,330	4%
	75 & older	285,000	83,510	29%	20,550	7%
	85 & older	70,000	31,670	45%	9,340	13%
TX	55 & older	3,313,000	464,330	14%	87,500	3%
	65 & older	1,915,000	351,140	18%	71,030	4%
	75 & older	811,000	228,310	28%	51,050	6%
	85 & older	203,000	87,930	43%	23,520	12%

APPENDIX: ESTIMATED RATES OF VISUAL IMPAIRMENT AMONG OLDER AMERICANS

State	Age Range	State Population (1995)	Nonsevere Visual Impairment (including severe) Number	Rate	Severe Visual Impairment (including blindness) Number	Rate
UT	55 & older	293,000	26,310	9%	4,590	2%
	65 & older	172,000	20,130	12%	3,760	2%
	75 & older	76,000	13,380	18%	2,750	4%
	85 & older	18,000	4,920	27%	1,220	7%
VA	55 & older	1,261,000	162,060	13%	31,380	2%
	65 & older	737,000	122,980	17%	25,510	3%
	75 & older	309,000	79,120	26%	18,140	6%
	85 & older	72,000	28,720	40%	7,940	11%
VT	55 & older	116,000	11,190	10%	2,010	2%
	65 & older	71,000	8,820	12%	1,690	2%
	75 & older	32,000	6,000	19%	1,260	4%
	85 & older	9,000	2,540	28%	630	7%
WA	55 & older	1,038,000	96,990	9%	17,370	2%
	65 & older	628,000	75,620	12%	14,440	2%
	75 & older	283,000	50,910	18%	10,660	4%
	85 & older	68,000	18,960	28%	4,770	7%
WI	55 & older	1,097,000	110,140	10%	19,460	2%
	65 & older	683,000	87,730	13%	16,480	2%
	75 & older	320,000	60,740	19%	12,470	4%
	85 & older	84,000	24,320	29%	5,940	7%
WV	55 & older	457,000	73,370	16%	15,730	3%
	65 & older	279,000	57,300	21%	13,080	5%
	75 & older	121,000	37,700	31%	9,480	8%
	85 & older	29,000	14,010	48%	4,230	15%
WY	55 & older	94,000	8,380	9%	1,400	1%
	65 & older	54,000	6,320	12%	1,140	2%
	75 & older	23,000	4,140	18%	820	4%
	85 & older	6,000	1,650	27%	390	6%

Source: American Foundation for the Blind, Department of Policy Research and Program Evaluation, New York, 1997, based on data from U.S. Bureau of the Census, *Model-Based Estimates of Specific Disabilities for States and Counties,* www.census.gov/hhes/www/disable.html (1997); and unpublished data from the 1993–94 Survey of Income and Program Participation, John M. McNeil, personal communication, February 1997.

MODULE 2

The Aging Eye: Age-Related Eye Conditions and Their Functional Implications

Vision is a complex sense involving the ability to see contrasts, detail, and the location of objects in the environment. Although the eye usually changes with age, natural changes in the healthy aging eye can be corrected by eyeglasses or contact lenses and their impact lessened by environmental modification. However, four eye conditions associated with the aging process—macular degeneration, glaucoma, diabetic retinopathy, and cataracts—may result in visual impairment. It is important that people who work with older individuals be able to recognize signs of vision loss to be able to help them get appropriate eye care and vision-related services.

Topic Outline

2.1 Normal Age-Related Changes in the Eye and Visual Functioning

    2.1.1 Reduced Visual Acuity

    2.1.2 Loss of Accommodation: Presbyopia

    2.1.3 Floaters

    2.1.4 Dry Eyes

- 2.1.5 Increased Need for Light
- 2.1.6 Difficulty with Glare
- 2.1.7 Difficulty with Adaptation to Light and Dark
- 2.1.8 Reduced Contrast Sensitivity
- 2.1.9 Reduced Color Perception
- 2.1.10 Reduced Depth Perception

2.2 Eye Conditions Associated with Aging
- 2.2.1 Macular Degeneration (Age-Related Maculopathy)
- 2.2.2 Glaucoma
- 2.2.3 Diabetic Retinopathy
- 2.2.4 Cataracts
- 2.2.5 Vision Loss Resulting from Stroke

2.3 Functional Aspects and Current Treatment of Vision Loss
- 2.3.1 Impact of Macular Degeneration on Visual Functioning
- 2.3.2 Treatment of Macular Degeneration
- 2.3.3 Impact of Glaucoma on Visual Functioning
- 2.3.4 Treatment of Glaucoma
- 2.3.5 Impact of Diabetic Retinopathy on Visual Functioning
- 2.3.6 Treatment of Diabetic Retinopathy
- 2.3.7 Impact of Cataracts on Visual Functioning
- 2.3.8 Treatment of Cataracts

2.4 Signs and Symptoms of Vision Loss

2.5 Dual Sensory Impairments: Vision and Hearing Loss

2.6 Vision Terminology
- 2.6.1 Low Vision
- 2.6.2 Severe Visual Impairment
- 2.6.3 Legal Blindness
- 2.6.4 Definitions of Visual Functioning

2.7 Eye Care and Low Vision Services
- 2.7.1 The Role of Eye Care Specialists
- 2.7.2 The Low Vision Evaluation
- 2.7.3 Types of Low Vision Devices
- 2.7.4 Reactions to Low Vision Devices
- 2.7.5 Low Vision Rehabilitation

**MODULE 2:
THE AGING EYE:
AGE-RELATED EYE CONDITIONS
AND THEIR FUNCTIONAL
IMPLICATIONS**

2.8 Need for Increased Awareness of Low Vision Services

　2.8.1 Making Referrals to Low Vision Services

　2.8.2 The Role of Service Providers in the Aging Network

2.9 Eye Care in Nursing Homes

Learner Objectives

1. The student will be able to describe the normal changes in the eye and visual functioning associated with aging.

2. The student will be able to identify the four leading eye conditions associated with the aging process and their functional implications for carrying out routine daily tasks.

3. The student will be able to describe the kinds of treatment currently available for each of the eye conditions.

4. The student will be able to define basic vision terms and understand how various types of vision loss affect everyday functioning.

5. The student will be able to identify the signs of vision loss.

6. The student will be able to describe the components of a functional low vision assessment and the low vision optical (and nonoptical) devices available to enable people who are visually impaired to make the best use of their remaining vision.

2.1 Normal Age-Related Changes in the Eye and Visual Functioning

Vision consists of the complex combination of visual acuity, color sense, the ability to distinguish contrasts, and the ability to evaluate the location of objects in the environment (space). Most older people experience normal changes in their eyes that are associated with the aging process. In addition, there are four major age-related eye conditions that may result in visual impairment. Before examining the specifics of these eye conditions, it is important to understand the normal changes that occur in the eye and in visual functioning associated with the aging process.

Changes in vision among older persons are the result of anatomic changes associated with the older eye. Examples of normal vision changes associated with aging are described in the following sections.

In general, environmental conditions such as adequate lighting, elimination of glare, and the use of color contrast are more significant for the visual functioning of older persons than of younger persons. Many of these helpful environmental modifications are minor and inexpensive; they can be made quite easily within the homes of older persons who are visually impaired, as well as in public environments.

2.1.1 Reduced Visual Acuity

Visual acuity is the ability to see objects clearly, and is measured by the high-contrast acuity charts typically found in an eye care professional's office. A visual acuity of 20/20 means that an individual reading the chart at 20 feet can see what the average person can at that distance; likewise, visual acuity of 20/40 means that the individual can see at 20 feet what the average individual can see at 40 feet.

Visual acuity generally declines modestly beyond age 60. For example, a reduced visual acuity of 20/30 or 20/40 with the best possible correction by eyeglasses, compared to a prior visual acuity of 20/20, is typical for an individual age 60 or older.

2.1.2 Loss of Accommodation: Presbyopia

Accommodation refers to focusing power—the ability to adjust the focus of the eyes as the distance between the individual and the object shifts. Loss of accommodation, or *presbyopia*, is the eye's decreasing capacity to focus at close range. People with presbyopia frequently hold reading materials at arm's length in order to get the print in focus.

The decrease in accommodation with age is caused by the hardening of the lens of the eye and by the change in muscle tone. Because the loss of the ability to see close objects or small print happens gradually over a lifetime, presbyopia is not typically noticeable until after age 40. Some people with presbyopia experience headaches or "tired eyes" while reading or doing other close work.

Presbyopia is correctable by bifocals, trifocals, reading glasses, or continuous-range glasses.

2.1.3 Floaters

Floaters are tiny spots or specks that float across the field of vision. Most people notice floaters in well-lit rooms or outdoors on a bright day.

Floaters usually are normal, but in some cases they warn of eye problems such as retinal detachment, especially if they occur with light flashes. If an individual notices a sudden change in the type or number of spots or flashes, she or he should consult an eye care physician.

2.1.4 Dry Eyes

Dry eyes occur when tear glands do not make enough tears or make tears of poor quality. Dry eyes can be uncomfortable, causing itching, burning, or even some loss of vision. An eye doctor may suggest using a humidifier in the home or special eye drops ("artificial tears"). Surgery may be needed for more serious cases of dry eyes.

2.1.5 Increased Need for Light

The amount of light reaching the back of the eye commonly decreases with age as a result of a smaller pupil and increased density or haziness associated with the older lens of the eye.

On average, an older person requires four times more light than a younger person. An individual age 80 and older requires 10 times more light than the average 25-year-old. However, the right amount of light for an older person with an age-related eye condition is a very individualized need.

Vision is typically good among older persons under conditions of optimal lighting. Optimal lighting conditions include more than one light source in a room, higher wattage light bulbs, and a light source directed onto the reading material or other materials.

2.1.6 Difficulty with Glare

Even though an older person typically needs much brighter light, vision can be reduced by too much *glare*, bright light that either shines directly or reflects into the eye.

Glare is caused by bright light reflecting from shiny surfaces or when a visual impairment causes light entering the eye to "bounce around" rather than to come into focus. An extreme adverse reaction to bright light and glare is referred to as *photophobia*.

The presence of glare increases difficulty in distinguishing objects from their background in the environment and in identifying faces. The older person's ability to recover from glare or from bright lights commonly decreases after age 50 as a result of changes in the lens and in retinal sensitivity.

Common sources of glare include highly polished floors, metal objects, mirrors, tiled or enameled floors and walls, and shiny table tops such as glass. The natural environment can also produce a great deal of glare that inhibits visual discrimination among older persons. Glare is caused outdoors by sunlight and indoors by sunlight streaming through a window onto a shiny surface or by fluorescent lighting. High-gloss paper such as that used in many magazines can also cause problems with glare and make reading extremely difficult.

Incandescent lighting is frequently more comfortable for the eye than fluorescent lighting. Incandescent lighting is better for spot lighting on close-up tasks, while fluorescent lighting is better for ambient illumination. A combination of both types of lighting can be most helpful for many older people.

More light that is properly directed, such as the use of a higher wattage light bulb, and properly arranged light sources throughout the room, especially a light source shining directly on a work area or reading area, are generally very helpful to the older individual. Increased wattage lighting, however, can cause glare or other discomfort for some older people. An individual approach to determining correct lighting is therefore extremely important.

2.1.7 Difficulty with Adaptation to Light and Dark

Adaptation to light and dark is the ability of the eyes to adapt to different levels of illumination. This involves the *rods* and *cones*, the photoreceptor cells of the retina. The rods, which contain the pigment rhodopsin, are sensitive to the presence of light and motion. The cones contain three different photopigments and give us the sense of color and fine detail.

At night, the rods are used to detect the movement of shapes in dim light. If lights are turned on, the eyes need time to adapt to the higher level of illumination, and the pigments of the cone cells are activated.

The eye adapts much more quickly from dark to light than from light to dark because of the speed with which the pigments can be restored.

The ability to adapt to darkness decreases significantly with age, and the time it takes to adapt to changing environments, from light to dim and from dim to light, increases as a result of changes in pupil size, the lens, and the retina. Familiar examples of these changing environments include going from outdoors into a movie theater, or from a restaurant to outdoors.

Individuals who have very limited visual fields, as in advanced glaucoma, have extremely limited functional vision in dim lighting.

2.1.8 Reduced Contrast Sensitivity

Contrast between light and dark is produced by the amount of light that is reflected from various surfaces: a light object is brighter than a dark object, for example. The difference in light and dark makes objects that contrast with their background easier to see. The cells in the retina and the brain identify contrast and edges, not absolute light or dark. The ability to differentiate light from dark is essential to good visual functioning.

The ability to recognize faces and objects in the environment involves seeing contrast as well as textures and patterns.

Contrast is an essential element for reading. Sharp, crisp images with black print on a white or pale yellow page produce the best contrast.

Compared to younger people, older persons need sharper contrasts and sharper edges around an object in order to differentiate that object from its background.

2.1.9 Reduced Color Perception

The ability to identify color commonly diminishes with age, and certain vision problems also cause difficulty in distinguishing colors. Colors that are close to each other on the hue circle, such as blue and green or red and orange, are the most difficult to distinguish.

The use of contrasting colors in the physical environment can help an older person to move about the environment more easily and to identify objects in the environment. Examples include a dark-colored door or door frame against light-colored walls or a dark-colored switch plate against a light-colored wall; these contrasts enable the older individual with less vision to function more easily.

2.1.10 Reduced Depth Perception

Reduction in depth perception makes it difficult for the individual to determine how close or far away an object is and how high or low something is. Loss of depth perception makes steps and street curbs difficult to recognize and manage.

A decrease in contrast sensitivity is one factor that diminishes the older person's ability to perceive depth.

2.2 Eye Conditions Associated with Aging

The four leading eye conditions that are associated with aging are macular degeneration, glaucoma, diabetic retinopathy, and cataracts. A description of these conditions is presented in this section, followed in the next section by a description of how each eye condition affects visual functioning and available treatment, to give service providers information about what their older clients experience as a result of various eye conditions. Because many older people also experience impaired vision as a result of a stroke, a brief section on post-stroke vision problems is included.

Of these conditions, three are conditions of the retina: age-related macular degeneration, diabetic retinopathy, and retinal detachment. The *retina* is a thin lining on the back of the eye (see Figure 2.1). It is made up of cells that receive visual images and pass them on to the brain. Thus, retinal disorders are a leading cause of vision loss in the United States.

2.2.1 Macular Degeneration (Age-Related Maculopathy)

Macular degeneration is the most common eye condition and the leading cause of visual impairment among older persons.

Age-related macular degeneration (ARMD) is a degenerative condition of the *macula*, the area of the retina responsible for central vision, acute vision, and much of color vision.

The macula is a small area in the middle of the retina made up of millions of cells that are sensitive to light. The macula makes vision possible from the center part of the eye. Over time, ARMD can reduce the sharp vision needed to see objects clearly and to do common tasks such as driving and reading.

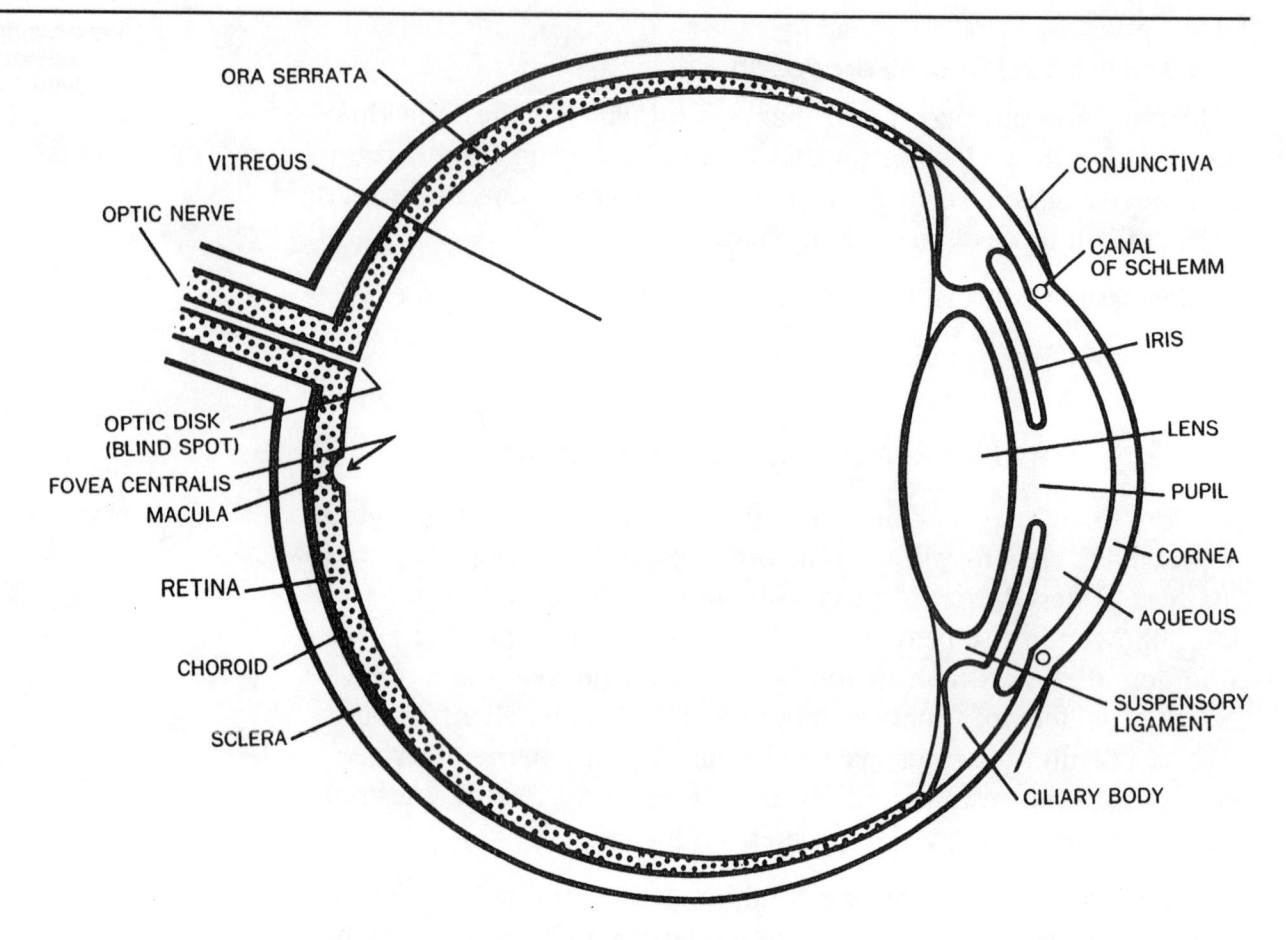

Figure 2.1. Cross section of the eye.

There are two types of ARMD: the *dry* or atrophic type, and the *wet* or hemorrhagic type. Dry ARMD is the more common form of macular degeneration. It is caused by the atrophy or thinning of the macula's tissue. Dry ARMD causes less severe vision loss than does the wet form.

Wet ARMD, the less common form, is called "wet" because in its advanced stages, it causes rapid growth of the small blood vessels beneath the retina. Affected blood vessels leak blood and other fluid, which form scar tissue. The result is more severe vision loss.

Macular degeneration is most frequently found among the Caucasian population.

2.2.2 Glaucoma

Glaucoma is an eye disease characterized by an increased level of intraocular pressure caused by the buildup of excess fluid in the eye. Glaucoma results in a loss of peripheral (side) vision. If undiagnosed and untreated, chronic elevated eye pressure can cause damage to or atrophy of the optic nerve. Once damage is done to the optic nerve, lost vision cannot be treated or restored.

The pressure of the fluid within the eye can be measured using special equipment in a procedure known as *tonometry*. Intraocular pressure is recorded in millimeters of mercury (mm Hg); normal pressure ranges from 12 to 22mm Hg.

A pressure check should be a routine part of a comprehensive eye examination for adults age 35 and older. An eye care professional can diagnose glaucoma before vision is lost by examining the optic nerve through a dilated pupil and by administering a visual field test.

There are three forms of glaucoma: congenital, primary, and secondary. The congenital form of glaucoma appears in young people, and secondary glaucoma is the result of injury or some form of trauma. Primary glaucoma is that form associated with the aging process. There are two types of primary glaucoma: open angle and closed angle.

Open-angle glaucoma is the type most frequently found in the United States, occurring in at least 90 percent of cases. It is usually detected in its early stages during a routine eye examination. It occurs when the eye's drainage canals gradually become clogged.

Closed-angle glaucoma, or acute glaucoma resulting from blockage of the angle between the iris and the cornea where fluid normally drains, usually has a sudden onset. It is characterized by pain in the eye, blurred vision, nausea, headaches, and rainbows around lights at night.

Onset of glaucoma is typically associated with age 40; the incidence of glaucoma increases among persons over 40 years old.

Glaucoma tends to run in families. The incidence of glaucoma is considerably higher among African-Americans than in the Caucasian population. African-Americans have a five times greater risk for glaucoma, and their rate for blindness resulting from glaucoma is roughly six times greater (National Advisory Eye Council, 1993). Therefore, it is critical that African-Americans have routine eye examinations that include a glaucoma check.

Individuals with diabetes or who are very nearsighted are at a higher risk of developing glaucoma. Individuals who have had eye surgery or injuries or who have used steroid medications for extended periods of time also may be at higher risk than the average person.

Glaucoma is especially dangerous because it often progresses without pain or obvious symptoms. This is why it is sometimes referred to as the "sneak thief of sight." Vision loss resulting from damage to the optic nerve is irreversible, but it is preventable if detected early and if treatment is started immediately.

2.2.3 Diabetic Retinopathy

Diabetic retinopathy occurs when small blood vessels stop feeding the retina properly. In its early stages, the blood vessels may leak fluid in the retina, which can affect the macula, the entire retina, or the vitreous (the clear, gel-like substance that fills the interior of the eye) and can distort vision. In the later stages of diabetic retinopathy, new vessels may grow and send blood into the center of the eye, causing serious vision loss.

Diabetic retinopathy is associated with diabetes, both type I (insulin dependent) and type II (commonly non-insulin dependent).

People with diabetes are more likely to lose vision from retinopathy, as well as from cataracts or glaucoma. About 40 percent of people with diabetes have at least mild retinopathy. Incidence increases with the disease's duration and when blood glucose cannot be controlled.

Diabetic retinopathy is associated with high blood pressure and poor control of blood sugar levels. Control of blood sugar levels and high blood pressure may deter the progression of diabetic eye disease, although it does not necessarily prevent it.

Individuals who are Hispanic, African-American, and Native American are most likely to develop diabetes. Individuals with these ethnic heritages should have routine medical and eye care at regular intervals, preferably annually.

2.2.4 Cataracts

Cataracts are cloudy areas in part or all of the lens of the eye. A healthy lens is clear and lets light through. Cataracts prevent light from passing easily through the lens, which causes loss of vision. Most cataracts form slowly and cause no pain, redness, or tearing in the eye.

Cataracts are characterized by a mild yellowing or cloudiness of the lens of the eye. In a young person, the lens is crystal clear, allowing light to pass through and focus on the retina.

As the lens ages, the nucleus or center of the lens turns yellow and loses its ability to accommodate (focus for close work), although the lens usually remains clear. As the lens continues to age, the nucleus turns from yellow to amber and ultimately to brown. This change in the color of the nucleus is almost universal in older persons.

A cataract is not significant, however, until it interferes with vision. Although cataracts result in diminished acuity because of the opacification of the lens, they do not affect a particular portion of the field of vision.

Some cataracts stay small and do not change eyesight significantly. If a cataract becomes large or dense, it usually can be removed by surgery.

2.2.5 *Vision Loss Resulting from Stroke*

Vision loss can be caused by a cerebral stroke, depending on the area of cortical involvement. It is one of the causes of vision loss seen most frequently by professionals serving older people, although it is not the result of an eye condition.

Just as a stroke may involve one side of the body, a defect of the optic pathways in the brain can result in *hemianopia,* or vision loss in half the visual field. Hemianopia in either brain hemisphere can affect reading. The affected individual may have difficulty finding the beginning of lines of text if vision loss is on the left; it may be difficult to see the ends of words if vision loss is on the right.

The individual with hemianopia may consistently bump into objects on the affected side and must learn to make good use of remaining vision associated with the unaffected hemisphere.

2.3 Functional Aspects and Current Treatment of Vision Loss

Because, as noted, vision is a complex sense made up of the ability to see both contrasts and detail and to evaluate the location of objects in the environment, age-related eye conditions affect vision in a variety of ways.

MODULE 2:
THE AGING EYE:
AGE-RELATED EYE CONDITIONS
AND THEIR FUNCTIONAL
IMPLICATIONS

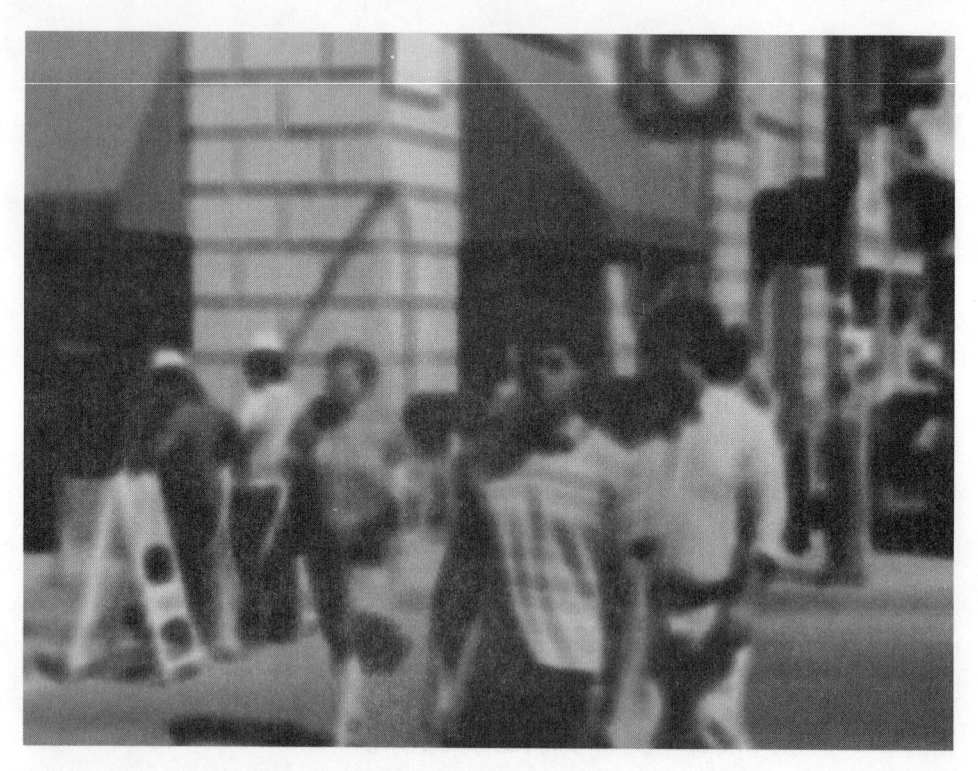

Overall blurred vision may be caused by cataracts, scars on the cornea, or diabetic retinopathy.

Although the eye usually changes with age, vision loss should not be accepted simply as a natural part of the aging process. Changes in vision are mildest in healthy aging eyes and can be corrected by eyeglasses or contact lenses.

Individuals experiencing age-related vision loss have difficulty with one or more of the following types of problems:

- *overall blurred vision*, which can be caused by cataracts, scars on the cornea, or diabetic retinopathy
- *loss of central or center vision*, frequently caused by macular degeneration
- *loss of peripheral or side vision*, most commonly caused by glaucoma or stroke

Each of the four leading eye conditions affects an individual's visual field functioning in different ways.

In addition to the medical treatments described in this section, many people with vision loss can enhance their visual functioning by using low vision devices. These are discussed later in this module.

2.3.1 Impact of Macular Degeneration on Visual Functioning

The major functional implications of macular degeneration are blurred or distorted central vision, central blind spots called *scotomas*, loss of detail vision, distortions of vision, and sometimes distortions in color vision. This condition develops very gradually in the atrophic forms and suddenly when subretinal vessels bleed or leak fluid.

Symptoms of macular degeneration are relatively easy to detect and include

- blurry areas on pages of text;
- wavy or bent appearance of straight lines on a page; and
- dark or empty spaces blocking the center area of the visual field.

Vision can be poor for reading or close handwork. Faces are difficult to recognize when someone is right in the center of the individual's visual field.

Despite loss of vision in the central field, peripheral vision remains good and generally intact. The individual with macular degenera-

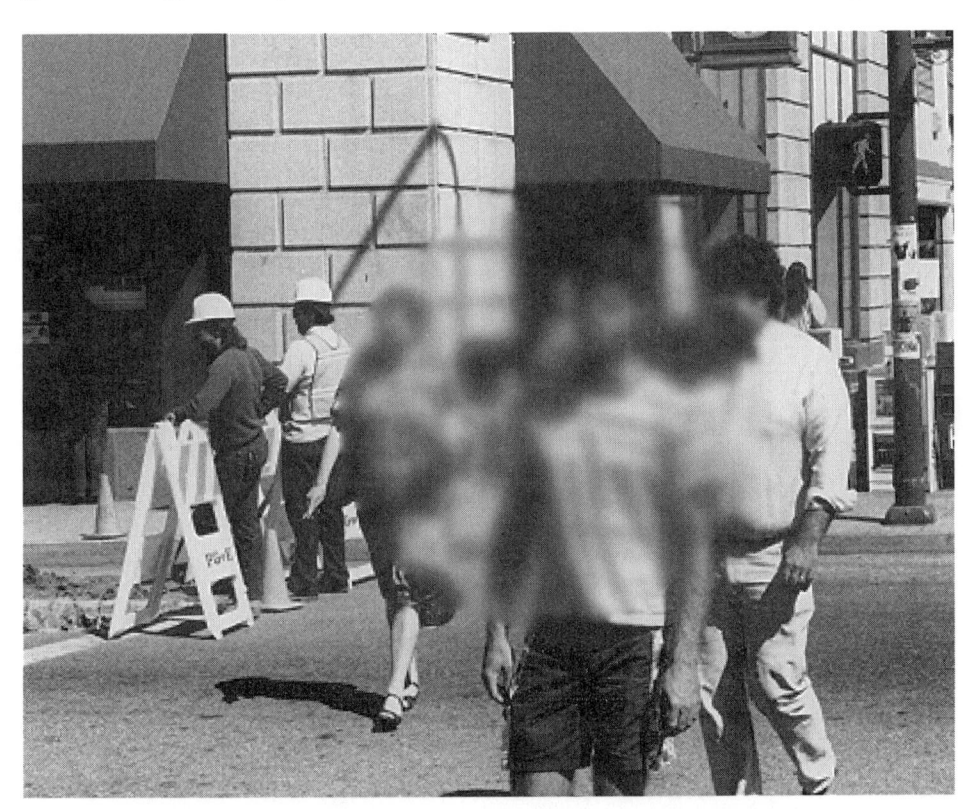

Loss of central or center vision is frequently caused by macular degeneration.

tion learns a technique called *eccentric viewing* to move the blind spot out of the way and to use peripheral vision to see an object.

Older persons do not become totally blind solely from macular degeneration.

Low vision devices, including various magnifiers and the closed-circuit television, prescribed by a low vision specialist frequently can enable the individual with macular degeneration to read and do other close work.

2.3.2 Treatment of Macular Degeneration

ARMD can be detected during an eye examination by the appearance of yellowish deposits at the back of the eye called *drusen*. The drusen do not necessarily interfere with visual acuity but are a symptom of the onset of ARMD.

In many cases, ARMD can be detected by a self-test using an Amsler grid. (It is important to note that self-testing with the Amsler grid is not a substitute for a regular eye examination, nor for a more complete visual field analysis in an eye care physician's office. It can, however, be used by an older person between routine examinations to detect signs of ARMD.)

The Amsler grid is a symmetrical pattern of squares with a central dot (see Figure 2.2). Changes in the appearance of the pattern that are noted with each eye signal macular degeneration or other forms of defects in the visual pathway.

The grid is placed on the wall at eye level or can be held by hand about 12 inches away from the individual or at the individual's distance for normal reading material. The individual should keep both eyes open and identify the black dot in the center. Then, while covering one eye, the individual looks at the dot in the center of the grid, testing one eye at a time. If the lines around the center dot are wavy, broken, blurred, or distorted in any way, this may be a sign of a macular problem.

The exact cause of macular degeneration is not known yet, although cigarette smoking is associated with increased risk for ARMD. There is no cure for macular degeneration. If detected early, the wet form of ARMD may be treated with laser surgery, which may slow the rate of vision loss. Blood vessels can be eliminated with laser photocoagulation if they have not extended beneath the

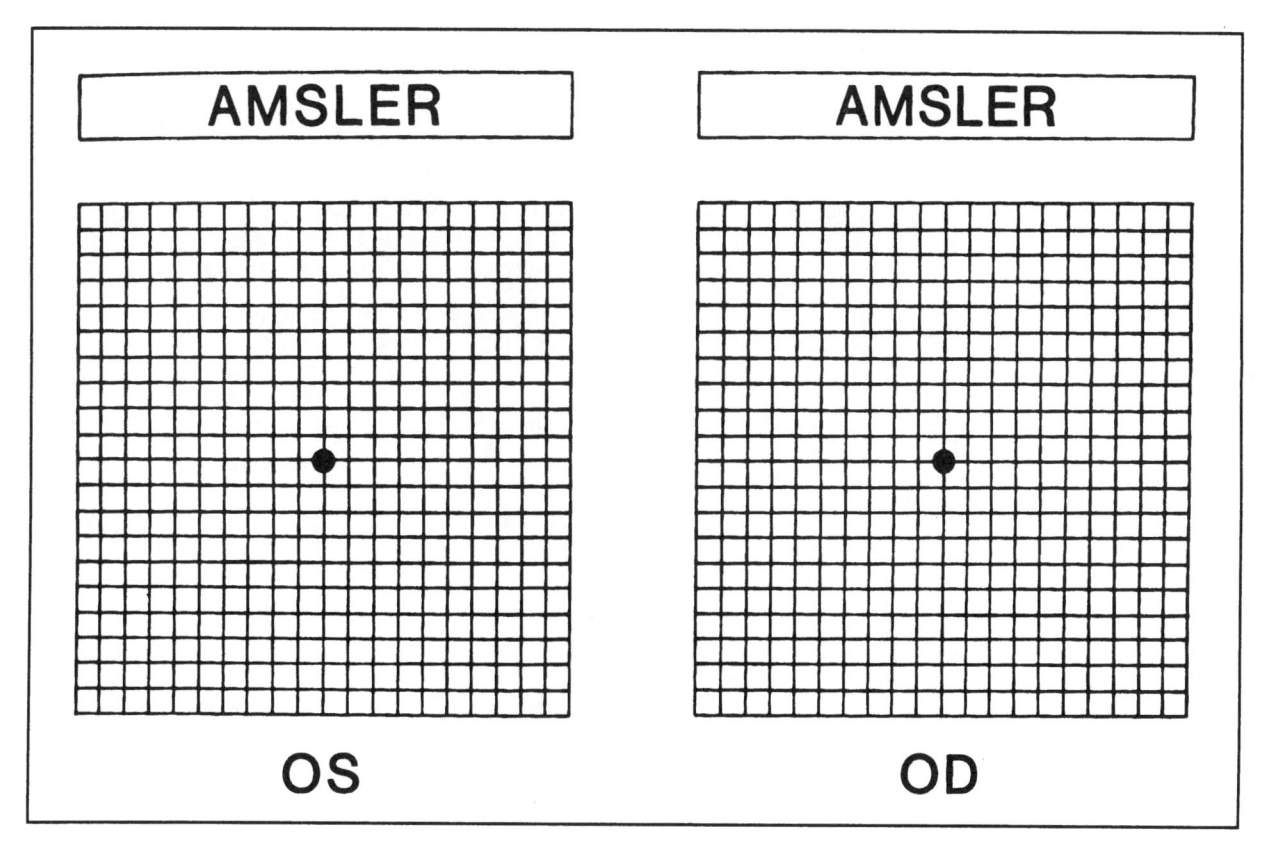

Figure 2.2. The Amsler grid can be used to detect changes in central vision.

fovea (the center of vision). This laser treatment can help in some severe cases, but it does not prevent recurrence.

2.3.3 Impact of Glaucoma on Visual Functioning

Glaucoma results in the loss of *peripheral vision* (side vision). Some signs and symptoms associated with glaucoma include

- inability to adjust the eyes to darkened rooms;
- frequent changes in eyeglasses without improved results;
- appearance of rainbow-colored rings around lights;
- blurred or foggy vision; and
- loss of side vision.

Individuals with glaucoma need to turn their heads from side to side in order to see everything around them, such as someone standing next to them.

Feeling safe and comfortable when walking becomes difficult. Loss of side vision may cause the individual to knock things over

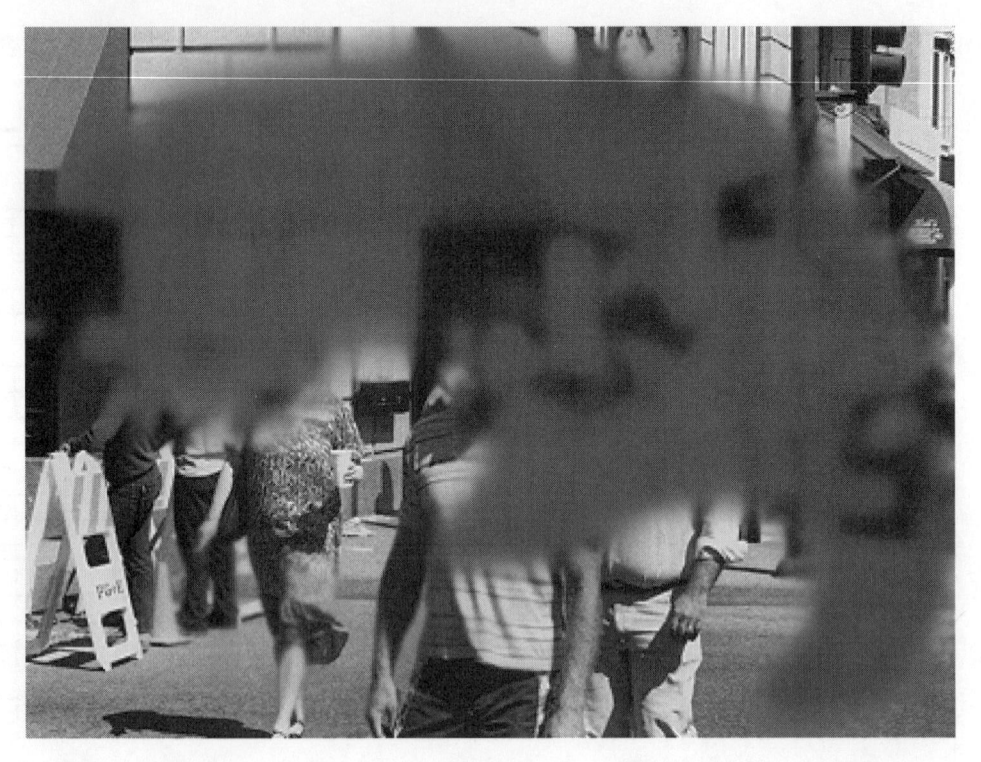

Loss of peripheral or side vision may be caused by untreated glaucoma or by a stroke.

accidentally or bump into things. Individuals with glaucoma may gradually lose some of their peripheral vision without realizing it.

2.3.4 Treatment of Glaucoma

If detected early, glaucoma is treatable with special eye drops that lower the pressure in the eye. Treatment also may include medication or surgery, both of which can have high success rates when glaucoma is detected early.

If eye drops are not effective, there is medication to reduce the level of fluid in the eye, but it has side effects. Laser surgery also is used to regulate eye pressure. If the progression of glaucoma is not halted by these methods, a surgical procedure to create an artificial outlet for fluid from the eye is recommended in some cases. This procedure is known as a filtering operation.

2.3.5 Impact of Diabetic Retinopathy on Visual Functioning

Diabetic retinopathy results in poor vision for reading; it causes print to be distorted or blurred. Many people with diabetic retinopathy experience increased sensitivity to glare.

The most common diabetes-related eye symptoms are

- changes in refraction, variable vision, or focus;
- blurred or hazy vision;
- sensitivity to glare;
- faulty color vision; and
- blindness.

Diabetes also increases a person's tendency to develop cataracts.

A complication of diabetic retinopathy is hemorrhage from the blood vessels leaking into the vitreous. If it clouds the vitreous, light that normally passes from the lens through the vitreous to the retina is blocked and vision is reduced.

2.3.6 Treatment of Diabetic Retinopathy

Retinopathy associated with diabetes cannot be prevented. If warning signs are present, visual problems associated with the condition can be prevented if examined and diagnosed at the earliest possible time. If untreated, diabetic retinopathy can result in total blindness.

If the presence of blood in the vitreous does not clear up over time, a *vitrectomy*, or surgical removal of the vitreous, can be performed. Blood and scar tissue are removed, and the vitreous is replaced with a clear solution.

In many cases, laser treatment can restore vision, stabilize it, or at least delay severe vision loss. When the leaking is caused by the growth of fragile new blood vessels, a type of laser treatment called *panretinal photocoagulation* can seal off leaking vessels and destroy abnormal ones. It is very important that a person with diabetes have an eye exam through dilated pupils every year.

2.3.7 Impact of Cataracts on Visual Functioning

Patients with cataracts experience decreased visual acuity; that is, more difficulty seeing in poorly lit environments, as a result of decrease in sensitivity to contrast. Many people with cataracts also experience increased sensitivity to glare. Print appears hazy and contrast is limited.

Approximately 50 percent of Americans between the ages of 65 and 74, and 70 percent age 75 and older, have cataracts (Faye, Rosenthal, & Sussman-Skalka, 1995).

The following are common signs and symptoms of cataracts:

- Distance vision can be blurred, especially outdoors, but there is no eye pain.
- The affected person experiences double vision, or sees "ghost images."
- The affected person experiences sensitivity to glare, such as the reflection of light from metal on a car, road, or pavement, or light from fluorescent ceiling fixtures.
- Print appears faded and lacking in contrast and is difficult to read in dim light.
- Colors appear faded or changed in hue; for example, a blue may seem to be a shade of green, white may appear gray or beige, and yellow may appear white.
- Sunglasses may appear to reduce the person's vision.
- Frequent changes of glasses do not help the person's vision.

2.3.8 Treatment of Cataracts

Cataract surgery has a high success rate. Ninety-five percent of patients experience improved vision after surgery if there are no other eye conditions present.

During surgery, the physician removes the clouded lens and, in most cases, inserts a clear intraocular lens of appropriate power. Cataract surgery is generally quite safe; however, complications do result from cataract surgery in approximately 5 percent of cases. It is one of the most common surgeries performed in the United States.

Thick eyeglasses are no longer needed after surgery because of the implanted lens.

2.4 Signs and Symptoms of Vision Loss

It is important that professionals, paraprofessionals, and volunteers working with older people, as well as family members, be able to recognize the signs of vision loss, particularly the early signs of onset, in order to help older people obtain needed eye care and vision-related rehabilitation services.

Warning signs of potentially serious vision problems are

- sudden hazy or blurred vision;
- recurrent pain in or around the eyes;
- double vision;

- flashes of light;
- halos around lights;
- unusual sensitivity to light or glare;
- change in the color of the iris; and
- sudden development of persisting floaters.

When any of these symptoms are noticeable to the individual, a vision problem may already be at an advanced stage, and professional eye care should be sought promptly. These signs are not just normal changes resulting from aging.

Certain forms of behavior indicate that an individual may be experiencing vision loss. It is important to keep in mind that some of these signs, or combinations of signs, also may be symptomatic of other conditions associated with aging. But it is critical that vision-related problems be diagnosed—and that the signs not be misdiagnosed as symptoms of other age-related conditions. The most common misperception or incorrect assumption is that an aging person is experiencing age-related dementia, which also is manifested by various forms of disorientation and failure to recognize family members.

Be alert if an older person manifests any of the difficulties listed in "How to Recognize Vision Loss in Older People." If professionals or family members notice these forms of behavior, the older person should be encouraged to have an eye examination by an eye care professional. It is also a good idea to inquire about a referral for a low vision evaluation by a low vision specialist—either an optometrist or ophthalmologist who specializes in diagnosing and treating low vision.

Even if these forms of behavior are not manifested, it is important to encourage every older person to have regular, routine eye care, including dilation.

2.5 Dual Sensory Impairments: Vision and Hearing Loss

The incidence of hearing impairment is greater than that of visual impairment among older persons. Many older persons experience both vision and hearing loss, each to varying degrees. Between 25 and 40 percent of people age 65 and older are hearing impaired, and the prevalence increases to 70–80 percent for individuals in their 70s and 80s (Moss & Parson, 1986).

It is important to be sensitive to the social and communication needs of this population. They have to struggle to communicate with family members, service providers, physicians, and the general public and to maintain a social network and to participate in group activities. When their needs go unrecognized or unaddressed, older persons with hearing and visual impairments frequently withdraw because of the difficulties involved in remaining connected to others (Boone, Watson, & Bagley, 1994; see also the Recommended Readings in the Resources section).

How to Recognize Vision Loss in Older People

If an older person exhibits any of the following behavior in the course of his or her daily activities, he or she may be experiencing a loss of vision. It is important for that person to have an eye examination—preferably by a low vision specialist—to see if that is the source of the difficulties.

Performing Usual Activities

- changing the way that he or she reads, watches television, drives, walks, or performs hobbies—or discontinuing one or more of these activities
- squinting or tilting the head to the side in order to focus on an object
- showing difficulty identifying faces or objects
- showing difficulty locating personal objects, even in a familiar environment
- reaching out for objects in an uncertain manner
- having difficulty identifying colors and selecting clothing in unusual color combinations

Reading and Writing

- discontinuing an established practice of reading the mail, a newspaper, or books
- holding reading material very close to the face or at an angle
- writing less clearly or precisely and showing difficulty writing on a line
- finding lighting in a room inadequate for reading and other activities

Moving about in the Environment

- brushing against the wall while walking
- consistently bumping into objects
- having difficulty walking on irregular or bumpy surfaces
- going up and down stairs slowly and cautiously, even though he or she has no other physical limitations

Eating and Drinking

- showing difficulty getting food onto a fork
- having difficulty cutting food or serving from a serving plate
- spilling food off the plate while eating
- pouring liquids over the top of a cup or drinking glass
- knocking over liquids while reaching across the table for another item

To help an individual with impaired hearing to remain involved, background noise—including music, loud conversations, ringing telephones, and the hum from computers or other equipment—should be kept at a minimum. It is also important for other people to speak directly to the individual, to introduce themselves, and to avoid touching the individual before speaking.

2.6 Vision Terminology

This section provides definitions of terms that refer to various degrees of visual functioning and vision loss, as well as terms describing vision skills or abilities. A variety of terms have been used at various times to describe people who are visually impaired, including *visually handicapped, partially sighted,* and *severely visually impaired.* Most recently, the preferred term is *low vision.*

2.6.1 Low Vision

The term *low vision* is used to describe the visual functioning of someone for whom ordinary eyeglasses, contact lenses, medical treatment, or surgery cannot correct vision to within the normal range. Such vision loss affects one's ability to carry out routine tasks of daily living. In many cases, however, an individual with low vision still has some good, usable vision and can learn to make the best use of it.

Among older persons, low vision can result from the specific eye conditions discussed here—cataracts, macular degeneration, glaucoma, or diabetic retinopathy—or other eye conditions, or it can result from a stroke.

The individual with low vision may experience one or more of the three types of vision problems: *overall blurred vision,* which can be caused by cataracts, scars on the cornea, or diabetic retinopathy; *loss of central or center vision,* frequently caused by macular degeneration; and *loss of peripheral or side vision,* most commonly caused by glaucoma or stroke.

The special kind of eye examination performed to evaluate low vision and the special optical devices that may be prescribed to enable the individual to make the best use of residual vision are described later in this module.

2.6.2 Severe Visual Impairment

The term *severe visual impairment* is found in the literature of the vision field and has been used in the collection of data regarding older people with significant vision problems (see Module 1). Therefore, it requires discussion, although the term *low vision* is now used most frequently to describe the same population with similar types and degrees of limitations in visual functioning.

Severe visual impairment has been defined functionally in data collection surveys such as the Health Interview Survey conducted by the National Center for Health Statistics as the inability to read newspaper print (see Module 1). The term is also used to describe an individual whose vision loss is severe enough to interfere with the ability to carry out activities of daily living (such as bathing, eating, dressing, and moving around the house) and instrumental activities of daily living (such as preparing meals, shopping, doing housework, and the like). This definition has been used to describe the visual functioning of older people whose vision loss is severe enough for them to benefit from vision rehabilitation services with the goal of enabling them to live independently, even though their clinical measure of visual acuity may be higher than that of individuals who are defined as legally blind.

2.6.3 Legal Blindness

Legal blindness is defined as a visual acuity of 20/200 or less in the better eye with the best possible correction, or a visual field of no more than 20 degrees (of a normal field of 175 to 180 degrees).

During the Great Depression, the U.S. government asked the American Medical Association (AMA) to develop a definition of blindness that could be used to determine which people were in need of special services because of the degree of their visual impairments. The AMA definition was then incorporated into the Social Security Act of 1935.

According to the definition, an individual can be considered legally blind for one of two reasons: limitations in visual acuity or in the visual field (or both).

A visual acuity of 20/200 means than an individual with this acuity can see, at a distance of 20 feet, what someone with 20/20 vision can see at 200 feet.

Individuals who are declared legally blind have varying degrees of vision, ranging from the ability to read print to no vision at all.

It is important to note that an individual who is totally blind is included in the category of legally blind; however, the designation of legal blindness is *not* synonymous with total blindness. The term *total blindness* means having no visual acuity; it includes individuals who have only light perception.

It is also important to keep in mind that many individuals who are legally blind have some remaining usable vision and can benefit from low vision services and the use of low vision devices.

Many older people who have low vision or are severely visually impaired but are not legally blind may have considerable functional limitations and thus may benefit from vision-related rehabilitation services.

Federal funding for vision-related vocational rehabilitation services is used by state vocational rehabilitation agencies to serve clients who have employment as their rehabilitation goal. Legal blindness has been the eligibility criterion for these services.

Older people have sometimes been served under the category of "homemaker," for adults who require rehabilitation services to be able to maintain a home and care for themselves and others within the home. However, people of traditional working age were frequently given priority over older individuals. This meant that many older people were unable to obtain the services they needed to continue living and functioning independently.

However, state rehabilitation agencies serving older people can now use federal funds from the Title VII, Chapter 2 independent living program of the Rehabilitation Act (see Module 4) to serve individuals age 55 and older who are severely visually impaired, as well as those who are legally blind.

2.6.4 *Definitions of Visual Functioning*

There are a number of different aspects of visual functioning. Difficulty with any of them affects vision. *Visual acuity* is the ability to see objects clearly. Reading the letters on an eye chart measures how well or how poorly a person can see an object only at the specified distance—20 feet, for example.

The *visual field* is the entire area covered by an individual's vision when looking straight ahead, usually 175 to 180 degrees. It is important for individuals to be aware of objects in the periphery as well as in the center of the field of vision.

Visual perception is the total process responsible for the reception and understanding of visual information. *Form perception* is the ability to organize and recognize visual images as specific shapes. The shapes encountered, such as the shapes of letters and words, are remembered, defined, and recalled.

Visual fixation is the ability to aim the eyes accurately when looking at a stationary object, such as reading a line of print on a printed page. *Pursuit fixation* is the ability to follow a moving object with the eyes, such as reading a sign while driving or while on a bus in motion.

Binocular fusion is the brain's ability to gather information received from each eye separately to form a single fused image. Double vision is the result of the brain's inability to do this.

Convergence is the ability to turn the two eyes toward each other to look at close objectives. This skill is necessary for binocular fusion to occur.

Stereopsis is the result of binocular fusion, which enables the individual to judge the relative distance between two objects.

2.7 Eye Care and Low Vision Services

Individuals age 55 and older need annual eye examinations for early diagnosis of eye diseases and changes in visual functioning to prevent unnecessary loss of vision or total blindness.

Community-based vision screenings provide an important form of preventive eye care. A vision screening does not replace a professional eye examination, but it can help identify early signs of vision problems and refer individuals who are at risk for eye disease for further eye examinations.

During a vision screening, participants are asked questions about their medical history to detect risk factors. If a possible problem is detected, the participant is advised to make an appointment with an eye care professional.

2.7.1 The Role of Eye Care Specialists

It is critical that individuals age 55 and older have an annual eye examination by an ophthalmologist or optometrist for early detection of eye conditions or disease and treatment for the prevention of further damage to the eye. Individuals age 35 and older should be tested annually for glaucoma.

The *ophthalmologist* is a medical doctor who specializes in conditions of the eye. The ophthalmologist diagnoses and treats eye diseases, performs eye surgery, and prescribes corrective lenses. Some ophthalmologists specialize in low vision; however, many refer low vision individuals to optometrists who specialize in low vision.

The *optometrist* is a health care professional trained and state licensed to provide primary eye care services. These services include

- administering comprehensive eye health and vision examinations;
- diagnosing and treating eye diseases and vision disorders;
- detecting eye signs of general health problems;
- prescribing eyeglasses, contact lenses, low vision rehabilitation, and vision therapy;
- prescribing medications and performing certain surgical procedures; and
- counseling patients about their vision needs as related to their occupations, avocations, lifestyles, and surgical alternatives.

The optometrist holds the doctor of optometry (O.D.) degree.

2.7.2 The Low Vision Evaluation

The *low vision specialist* is an optometrist or ophthalmologist who has specialized training and certification in low vision. The low vision specialist conducts a low vision evaluation, determining the extent of the individual's use of remaining vision, and works with the patient to maximize the use of remaining vision.

Rosenbloom (1992) proposed the following five principles of low vision care of older adults.

- Distinguish between the effects of aging and disease.
- See the older individual as a whole person.
- Use a team approach.
- Emphasize the older person's visual goals.
- Improve the person's quality of life by facilitating independence and goal-directed activity.

**MODULE 2:
THE AGING EYE:
AGE-RELATED EYE CONDITIONS
AND THEIR FUNCTIONAL
IMPLICATIONS**

The components of the low vision evaluation are as follows:

1. comprehensive patient history
2. functional low vision assessment
3. prescription of optical devices for near and distance vision
4. instruction and adaptive training in the use of optical devices
5. follow-up care and retraining in the use of devices

The low vision evaluation can be an extremely positive and reinforcing experience for the older person who is experiencing a significant vision loss but still has usable remaining vision.

The clinical low vision evaluation determines whether an individual with low vision can benefit from optical and nonoptical devices and from adaptive techniques to enhance visual functioning. The low vision evaluation is an assessment of functional vision—that is, the individual's ability to use remaining vision in a variety of tasks

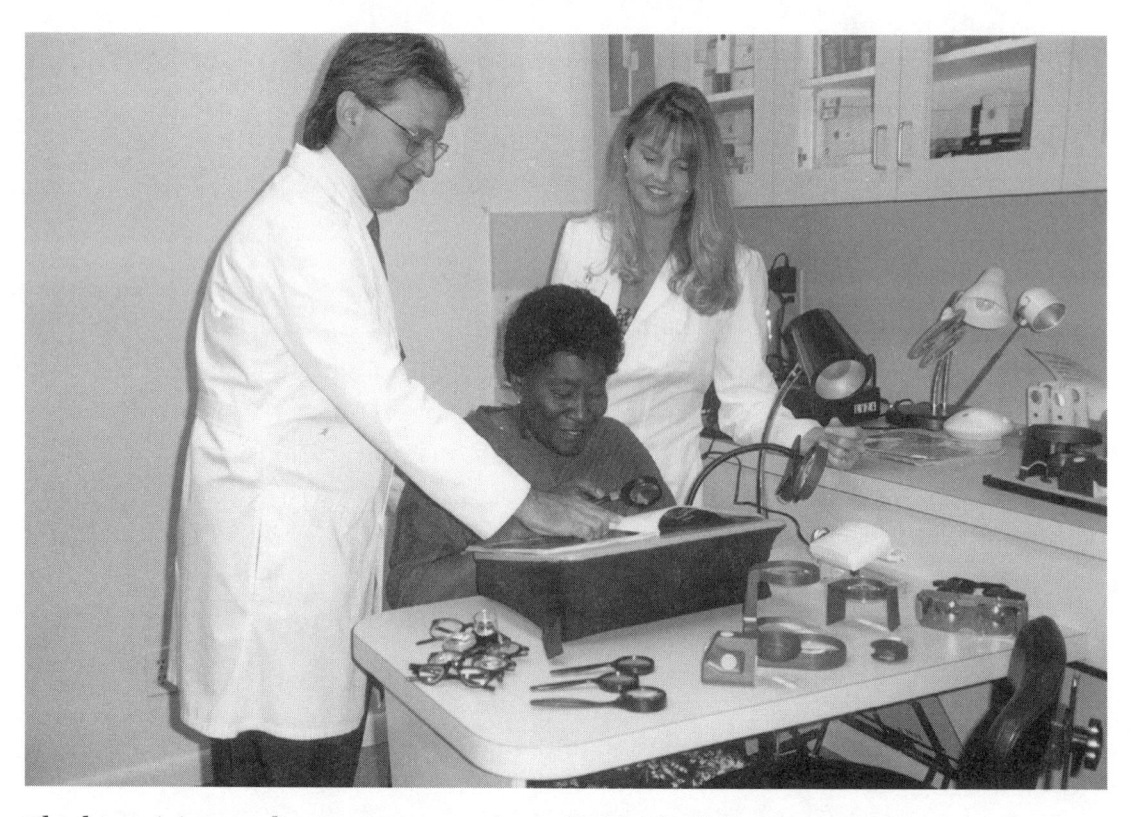

The low vision evaluation assesses the individual's functional vision and ways to maximize its use. Shown are a variety of handheld, stand, and lighted magnifiers and high-intensity lamps.

EYE CARE AND LOW VISION SERVICES

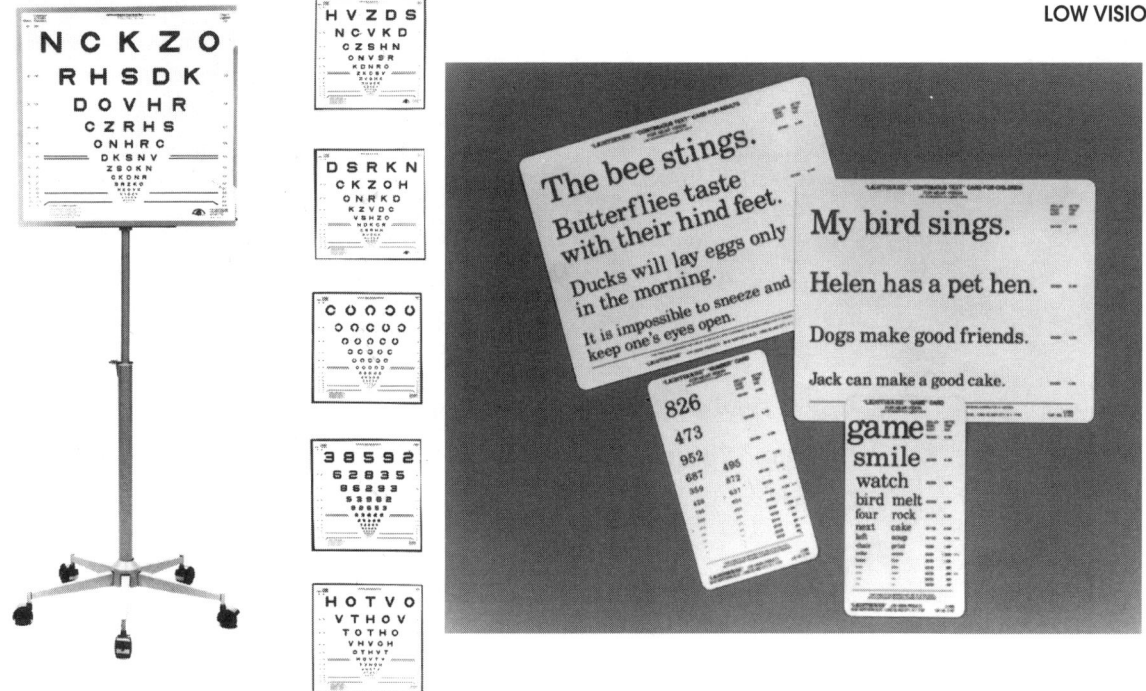

These Lighthouse distance (left) and near (right) visual acuity charts are commonly used to assess individuals with low vision.

and settings. It includes measures of near and distance vision, visual fields, eye movements, and responses to specific environmental characteristics such as light and color.

Low vision charts provide higher-contrast letters than standard eye charts and flexibility in the distance used during testing, such as the Lighthouse Distance Visual Acuity Chart, which is on wheels, and the large-print Lighthouse near-acuity cards.

The older person with usable functional vision experiences success during a low vision evaluation because the low vision specialist focuses on what the older person can see, rather than on his or her decreased acuity. The eye examination focuses on how to make the best use of that vision with the use of adaptive devices and under the best possible environmental circumstances.

The low vision specialist prescribes low vision devices to assist the individual in distance vision and close-up vision. The older person has the opportunity to work with several devices to determine which one works best for his or her remaining vision.

Next, the older person is allowed to borrow the devices and is encouraged to use them at home or in other environments in which the devices are needed for selected tasks or activities. Only after using the devices successfully in their own actual environments should patients with low vision receive or purchase them.

The low vision evaluation includes follow-up to ensure that the older person is continuing to use the devices successfully. If additional help is needed, follow-up instruction is provided.

2.7.3 Types of Low Vision Devices

Low vision devices are optical devices that are stronger than regular eyeglasses. They can help individuals with low vision make the best use of their remaining vision by magnifying, filtering light, or increasing the usable field of vision. Some examples of low vision devices include the following:

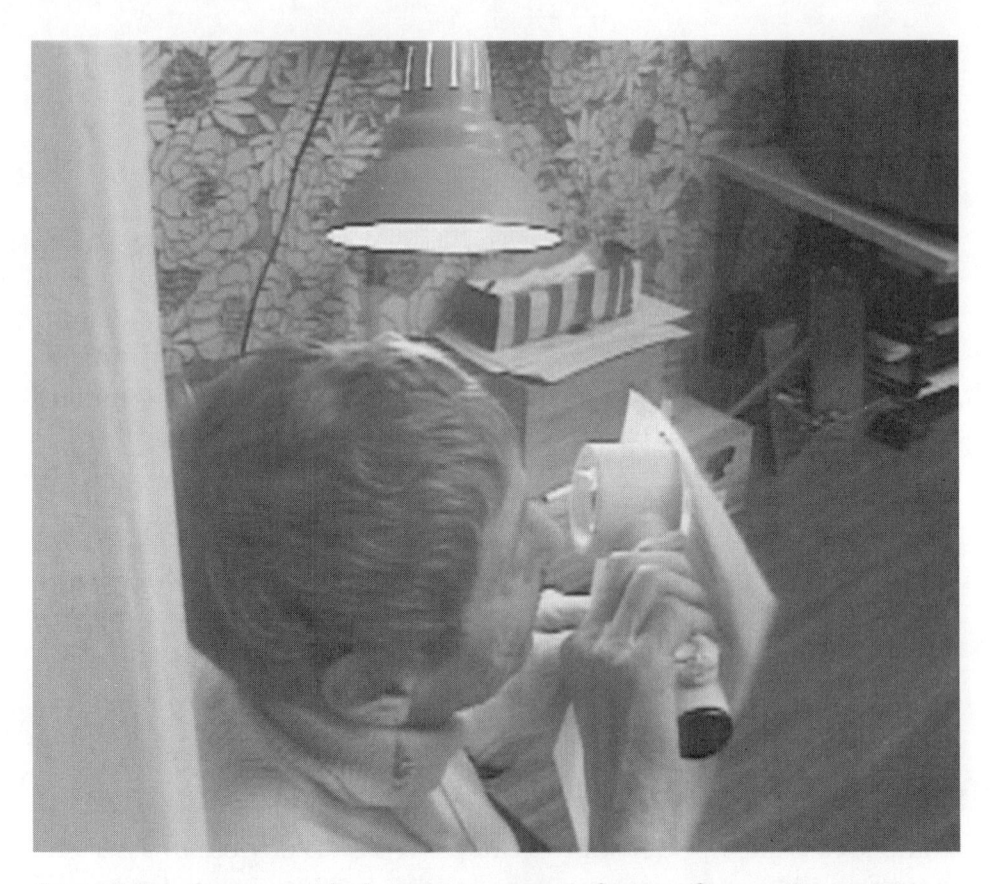

Low vision devices include various types of magnifiers, microscopes, and telescopes. This woman is reading her mail using a lighted hand-held magnifier and a high-intensity lamp.

**EYE CARE AND
LOW VISION SERVICES**

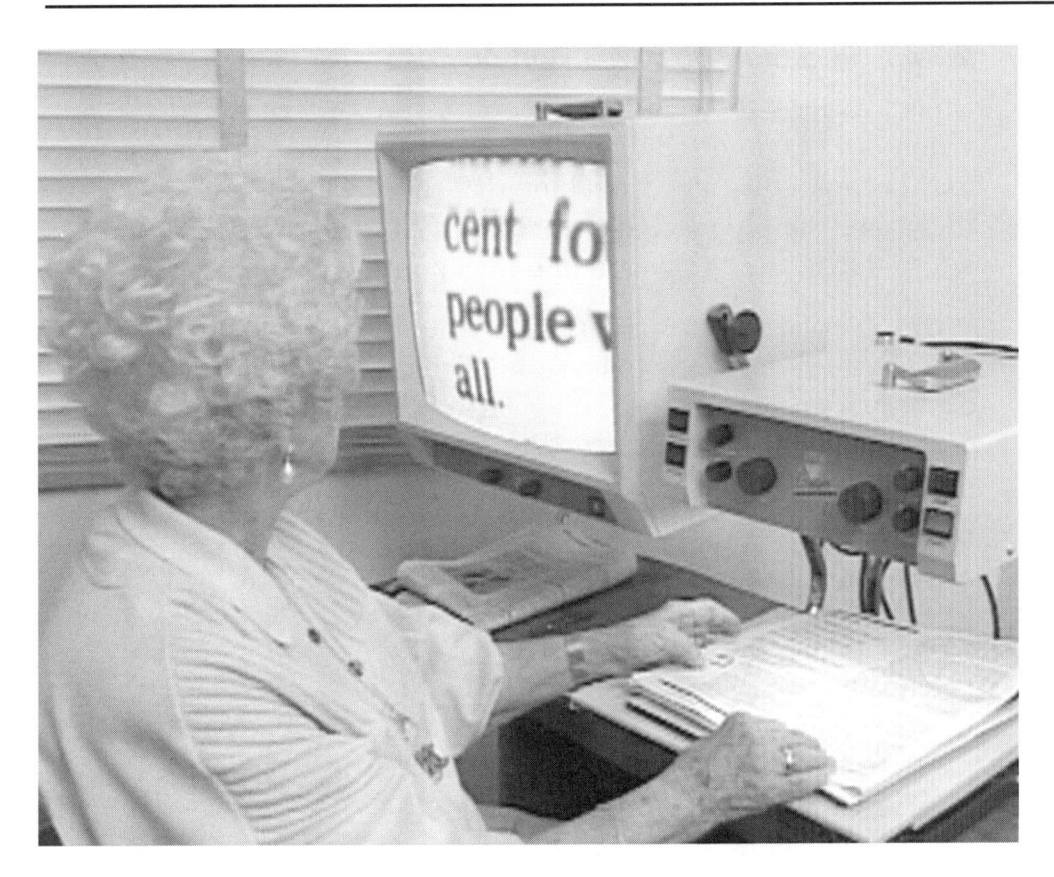

A closed-circuit television (CCTV) is a low vision device that uses video technology to magnify reading material.

- handheld or stand magnifiers and microscopic spectacles for reading print or performing other near tasks
- pocket-sized telescopes—handheld or frame mounted—for distance vision, such as reading a street sign or identifying the number of an approaching bus
- closed-circuit televisions (CCTVs) for reading, which magnify and project printed materials onto a television screen
- high-intensity lamps or other nonoptical devices to enhance vision for reading and other close-up tasks such as writing or sewing

Also available are high-tech devices, including these:

- computers with screen magnification
- large-print display software to attach to the computers
- portable video and electronic magnifiers for reading
- optical scanners that convert print into synthetic speech, such as the Kurzweil Personal Reader

2.7.4 Reactions to Low Vision Devices

Unless there is thorough instruction in the proper use of the low vision devices, and follow-up training when needed, older people may become frustrated, conclude that the device does not work for them, and simply place it in a drawer. This reaction is sometimes referred to as the "drawered phenomenon."

The older person's reactions to the introduction of both high-tech and low-tech devices is frequently related to the individual's previous experience with technology if technology was part of their vocational or avocational activities (Orr & Piqueras, 1991).

After low vision devices are prescribed and taken home, it is common for older people to reject them. Some of the reasons for this are the following (Watson, 1996, p. 379):

- further deterioration of vision
- declining health
- inability to adjust to the device because of a very close fixation distance, a small field of view, or a narrow depth of focus
- inadequate training or practice
- a change in the individual's visual goals that are not satisfied by the prescribed device
- differences between the ergonomics at the low vision clinic and the home setting, such as different lighting and seating or the lack of a reading stand or colored filters at home
- dizziness or nausea when first using the device
- psychosocial factors such as depression or anxiety, lack of support from family members or friends, cosmetic reasons, or fear of being vulnerable to crime in public

2.7.5 Low Vision Rehabilitation

Some individuals may benefit from vision-related rehabilitation services, in which professionals train the older person to use alternative methods to perform routine daily activities and to move about safely, both indoors and outside the home.

In addition to optical low vision devices, the person in low vision rehabilitation may learn to use such nonoptical devices as these:

- felt-tipped pens
- objects with tactile marking, such as a kitchen timer, watch, or board game
- sewing needles with large or hinged eyes and needle threaders

EYE CARE AND
LOW VISION SERVICES

- talking watches, clock, and calculators
- large-numeral telephone, clocks, timers, thermostats, and calculators
- large-print reading materials
- Talking Books (books on audiocassette provided by the Library of Congress)
- large-print or braille board games and playing cards
- writing guides such as a signature card, envelope-addressing guide, check template, or bold-lined paper

The term *low vision rehabilitation* is used to convey the broad scope and comprehensiveness of services available to the individual with low vision. The goal of low vision rehabilitation is to enable the individual with low vision to make the best use of his or her remaining vision to carry out routine daily tasks and ameliorate

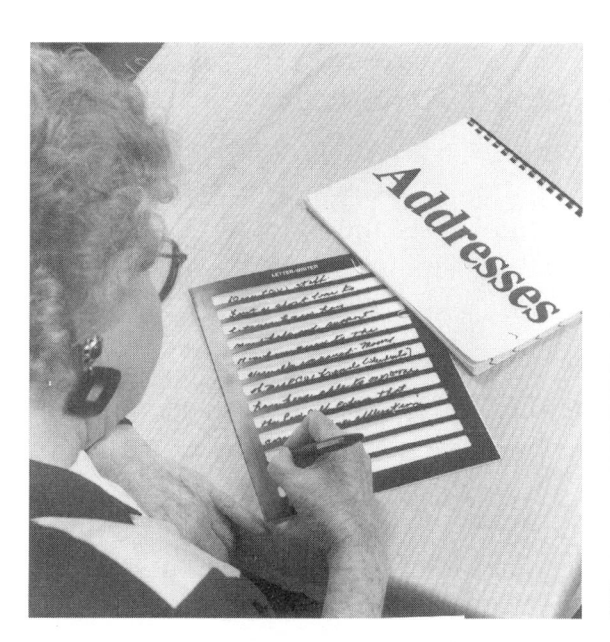

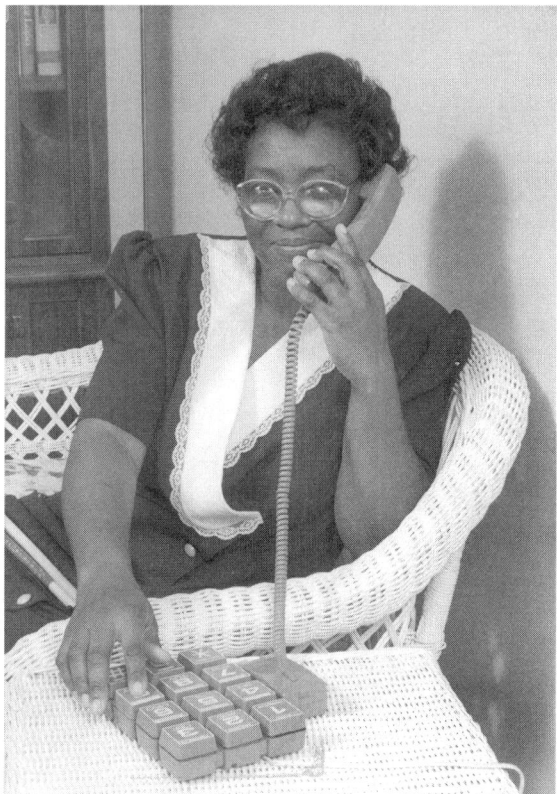

Through vision rehabilitation services, people with low vision learn to use such nonoptical assistive devices as writing guides with bold felt-tipped markers and large-print books (left) and telephones with large numerals (right).

functional disability. This process is described in more detail in Module 4.

2.8 Need for Increased Awareness of Low Vision Services

In spite of the critical role that low vision services can play, many older persons, their family members, and service providers have never heard of low vision services or assistive low vision devices. Even some physicians may not be fully acquainted with the value of low vision services or where they are available in the community.

Low vision services are located in the private offices of low vision specialists and at low vision clinics or centers. Low vision clinics may be free-standing or associated with a hospital, a college of optometry, or a vision-related rehabilitation agency serving blind and visually impaired persons.

The availability of low vision services across the country is growing, but low vision services are not available in every community. However, each state has affiliate offices of the American Optometric Association and the American Academy of Ophthalmology (see Resources), which can serve as referral sources. Each organization has a low vision section of specialists in low vision.

2.8.1 Making Referrals to Low Vision Services

Ophthalmologists and optometrists who are not specialists in low vision should refer low vision patients to a low vision specialist for a low vision evaluation. Ophthalmologists and optometrists can play a critical role in ensuring that individuals with vision loss learn to make the best use of their vision.

However, not all eye care professionals tend to make referrals beyond the medical arena, either for low vision assessment or for vision-related rehabilitation services. It is therefore essential for other professionals to know enough about low vision services to educate the older person and family members about their importance and to assist in the referral process (see Modules 4 and 5).

2.8.2 The Role of Service Providers in the Aging Network

Service providers in the aging network and other professionals outside the vision field would do well to ask any older person who is visually impaired the question, "Have you had a low vision evaluation by a low vision specialist?" Anyone who answers no should be referred to a low vision specialist.

The more that people know about the nature of the low vision evaluation and services, the more effective they can be in ensuring that older individuals get the low vision services and rehabilitation they need.

2.9 Eye Care in Nursing Homes

The level and frequency of eye care in nursing home settings varies tremendously across the country. On the average, residents have an eye examination every two years, and in some settings, every year. A number of studies have found, however, that there is no standard for eye care in nursing homes, that many nursing homes do not have a policy for screening residents' vision, and that the referral rate is not significantly higher for those residents who complain about their vision than for those who do not (Morse, O'Connell, Joseph, & Finklestein, 1988).

Linking nursing homes to eye care professionals, including low vision specialists, is critical if residents are to avoid unnecessary vision loss, and if they are to make the best use of remaining vision.

Low vision clinics need to reach out to the community and establish or expand the availability of mobile low vision services. They need to bring these services into nursing homes, adult residences, retirement communities, and other congregate facilities that serve older individuals.

Administrators of nursing homes, retirement communities, and other facilities serving older people are encouraged to reach out to the eye care community to bring services to the residents.

Increased awareness and knowledge of age-related eye conditions, their functional implications, and their treatment can enable older Americans to make the best use of their vision for independent living and productivity for as long as possible.

References

Boone, S. G., Watson, D., & Bagley, M. (Eds.). (1994). *The challenge to independence: Vision and hearing loss among older adults.* Little

Rock: University of Arkansas Rehabilitation Research and Training Center for Persons Who Are Deaf and Hard of Hearing.

Faye, E., Rosenthal, B. P., & Sussman-Skalka, C. J. (1995). *Cataract and the aging eye.* New York: The Lighthouse National Center for Vision and Aging.

Morse, A. R., O'Connell, W., Joseph, J., & Finklestein, H. (1988). Assessing vision in nursing home residents. *Journal of Vision Rehabilitation, 2*(4), 1–10.

Moss, A. J., & Parson, V. L. (1986). Current estimates from the National Interview Survey: United States—1985. *Vital and Health Statistics,* Series 10, No. 160 (DHHS Publication No. PHS 86-1588). Washington, DC: National Health Center for Statistics.

National Advisory Eye Council. (1993). *Vision research: A national plan, 1994–1998.* Bethesda, MD: National Eye Institute, National Institutes of Health.

Orr, A. L., & Piqueras, L. S. (1991). Aging, visual impairment and technology. *Technology and Disability, 1*(1),47–54.

Rosenbloom, A. A. (1992) Care of the visually impaired elderly patient. In A. A. Rosenbloom & M. W. Morgan (Eds.), *Vision and aging* (2nd ed.) (pp. 237–366). Stoneham, MA: Butterworth-Heinemann.

Watson, G. R. (1996). Older adults with low vision. In A. L. Corn & A. J. Koenig (Eds.), *Foundations of low vision: Clinical and functional perspectives* (pp. 363–394). New York: AFB Press.

RECOMMENDED TEACHING METHODS

Class Discussion

Explore with students their level of awareness about the four leading eye conditions associated with aging. Have students discuss these conditions for the first 5 to 10 minutes. Students may respond out of professional, personal, or family experience.

Lecture

Most of the content of this module is taught most effectively through lecture supported by videotapes or slides (see Resources), describing how individuals see with various eye conditions, to establish a basic knowledge base for students.

Videotape

Show the video *Not Without Sight* (1975), which demonstrates how individuals see who have one of the common eye conditions described in this module (see Resources section).

Guest Speakers

As resources and time allocation permit, the content of Module 2 can be covered effectively by a guest optometrist with a specialization in low vision or an ophthalmologist with similar specialization. These specialists can describe eye function and eye conditions, accompanied by slides, and they can also bring low vision devices for display, hands-on demonstration, and trial by students.

Experiential Exercises

Students can experience for themselves examples of what and how individuals with various eye conditions see by using low vision simulators, which approximate various eye conditions (see Resources section). A low vision specialist or a rehabilitation teacher from an agency serving people who are blind or visually impaired may be able to bring vision simulators and facilitate the experience.

Students can try walking around wearing the simulators, and they can attempt various tasks with the use of simulators and low vision devices. A frequently used technique for sensitivity training during in-service training sessions is to have participants eat a meal or walk with a sighted guide while wearing a blindfold or a vision simulator.

Field Trip

As time and resources permit, arrange for the class to visit a low vision clinic. To make the best use of the experience, students should visit a clinic that is part of an agency that provides an array of vision-related rehabilitation services. In addition to a presentation by a low vision specialist and hands-on experience with low vision devices, students would have the opportunity to become familiar with evaluation equipment and the testing environment.

MODULE 2: THE AGING EYE: AGE-RELATED EYE CONDITIONS AND THEIR FUNCTIONAL IMPLICATIONS

RESOURCES

Additional information about vision loss and the services provided by low vision specialists and vision rehabilitation specialists can be obtained from state rehabilitation agencies and local private agencies serving people who are blind or visually impaired. The state rehabilitation agency, private agencies, as well as low vision services and information and referral services in each state, can be found in the *Directory of Services for Blind or Visually Impaired Persons in the United States and Canada, 25th Edition,* published by AFB Press (1997). The sections on low vision services are especially useful.

Recommended Readings

Bagley, M. (1994). *Confident living program: A community-based learning experience for older adults with vision and/or hearing loss.* Sands Point, NY: Helen Keller National Center for Youths and Adults Who Are Deaf-Blind.

Bailey, I. L., & Hall, A. (1990). *Visual impairment: An overview.* New York: American Foundation for the Blind.

Corn, A. L., & Koenig, A. J., (Eds.). (1996). *Foundations of low vision: Clinical and functional perspectives.* New York: AFB Press.

Faye, E., Rosenthal, B. P., & Sussman-Skalka, C. J. (1995). *Cataract and the aging eye.* New York: Lighthouse National Center for Vision and Aging.

Faye, E., & Stuen, C. S. (1992). *The aging eye and low vision: A study guide for physicians.* New York: Lighthouse National Center for Vision and Aging.

Glaucoma Research Foundation. (1996). *Understanding and living with glaucoma: A reference guide for people with glaucoma and their families.* San Francisco: Author.

Lucey, H., Belser, D., & Glass, L. (1989). *Beyond refuge: Coping with losses of vision and hearing in late life.* Sands Point, NY: Helen Keller National Center for Youths and Adults Who Are Deaf-Blind.

Rosenbloom, A. A. (1992). Care of the visually impaired elderly patient. In A. A. Rosenbloom & M. W. Morgan (Eds.), *Vision and aging: General and clinical perspectives* (2nd ed.) (pp. 237–266). Stoneham, MA: Butterworth Press.

Rosenbloom, A. A. (1992). Physiological and functional aspects of aging, vision, and visual impairment. In A. L. Orr (Ed.), *Vision and aging: Crossroads for service delivery* (pp. 47–68). New York: American Foundation for the Blind.

Swanson M. (1994). Low vision and aging. In S. E. Boone, D. Watson, & M. Bagley (Eds.), *The challenge to independence: Vision and hearing loss among older adults* (pp. 73–92). Little Rock: University of Arkansas Rehabilitation Research and Training Center for Persons Who Are Deaf and Hard of Hearing.

Swanson, M. (1994). Vision changes with aging. In S. E. Boone, D. Watson, & M. Bagley (Eds.), *The challenge to independence: Vision and hearing loss among older adults* (pp. 61–72). Little Rock: University of Arkansas Rehabilitation Research and Training Center for Persons Who Are Deaf and Hard of Hearing.

Further Readings

Faye, E. E. (1984). *Clinical low vision* (2nd ed.). Boston: Little, Brown.

Genesky, S. M., & Zarit, S. H. (1992). Low vision care in a clinical setting. In A. A. Rosenbloom & M. W. Morgan (Eds.), *Vision and aging: General and clinical perspectives* (2nd ed.) (pp. 424–444). Stoneham, MA: Butterworth-Heinemann.

Jose, R. T. (1983). *Understanding low vision*. New York: American Foundation for the Blind.

Morgan, M. W. (1992). Normal age-related vision changes. In A. A. Rosenbloom & M. W. Morgan (Eds.). *Vision and aging: General and clinical perspectives* (2nd ed.) (pp. 178–199). Stoneham, MA: Butterworth-Heinemann.

Orr, A. L. (1997). Assistive technologies for older people who are visually impaired. In R. Lubinski & D. J. Higginbotham (Eds.), *Communication technologies for the elderly: Vision, hearing, and speech* (pp. 71–102). San Diego: Singular Publishing Group.

Schumer, R. A. (1997). Changes in vision and aging. In R. Lubinski & J. Higginbotham (Eds.), *Communication technologies for the elderly: Vision, hearing and speech* (pp. 41–70). San Diego: Singular Publishing Group.

Videotapes

Not without sight. (1975). New York: American Foundation for the Blind.

The 20-minute video *Not Without Sight* describes the major types of visual impairment, their causes, and their effects on vision. Camera simulations approximate what people with each of the common eye conditions described in this module actually see. The video also demonstrates how people with low vision make the best use of their remaining vision.

Other Materials

The functional vision screening questionnaire. (1996). New York: The Lighthouse.

The Functional Vision Screening Questionnaire is a screening tool that identifies older people who may be experiencing vision problems and who would benefit from seeing an optometrist or an ophthalmologist. The 15-item questionnaire is available in English, Spanish, Italian, German, French, Polish, and Chinese. It may be filled out independently by an older adult or administered by an interviewer. Details on scoring and interpreting the results are included. Each questionnaire is produced in pads of 25.

Eye Care and Vision Organizations

This listing includes a number of organizations that provide information and publications on normal eye changes, eye care, and eye diseases.

American Academy of Ophthalmology
P.O. Box 7424
San Francisco, CA 94120-7424
(800) 222-EYES (helpline)
http://www.aao.org

Publishes videotapes, audiotapes, slide-scripts, referral guidelines, newsletters, fact sheets, and programs. The National Eye Care Project has a helpline number that refers callers to local ophthalmologists who will provide free eye care to older people in need.

American Council of the Blind
1155 15th Street, N.W., Suite 720
Washington, DC 20005

(202) 467-5081 or (800) 424-8666
FAX: (202) 467-5085
E-mail: ncrabb@access.digex.net
http://www.acb.org

Promotes effective participation of people who are blind or visually impaired in all aspects of society. Acts as a national information clearinghouse. Provides information and referral; consumer advocate support; and consultative and advisory services to individuals, organizations, and agencies.

American Foundation for the Blind
11 Penn Plaza, Suite 300
New York, NY 10001
(212) 502-7600 or (800) 232-5463 or TDD (212) 502-7662
FAX: (212) 502-7777
E-mail: afbinfo@afb.org
http://www.afb.org

Serves as an information clearinghouse for people who are blind or visually impaired and their families, professionals, organizations, schools, and corporations. Publishes books, periodicals, and other materials for consumer and professional education. Maintains a World Wide Web site and operates a toll-free telephone information line. Maintains offices in Atlanta, Chicago, Dallas, and San Francisco, and a governmental relations office in Washington, DC.

American Optometric Association
243 North Lindbergh Boulevard
St. Louis, MO 63141
(314) 991-4100 or (800) 262-2210
FAX: (314) 991-4101
http://www.aoanet.org

Provides free consumer information materials on eye health and vision. Has a low vision section that provides consumer information and referrals.

Association for Macular Diseases
210 East 64th Street
New York, NY 10021
(212) 605-3719

Provides information and education on macular degeneration. Maintains support group for persons with macular degeneration and provides individual counseling by telephone and mail.

Better Vision Institute
Vision Council of America
1800 North Kent Street, Suite 904
Rosslyn, VA 22209
(703) 243-1508
FAX: (703) 243-1537
http://www.visionsite.org

Makes public aware of need for eye care. Publishes informational material and maintains library.

**The Foundation Fighting Blindness
(National Retinitis Pigmentosa Foundation)**
Executive Plaza 1, Suite 800
11350 McCormick Road
Hunt Valley, MD 21031-1014
(410) 785-1414 or TDD (410) 785-9687 or
(888) 394-3937 or TDD (800) 683-5551
FAX: (410) 771-7470
http://www.blindness.org

Serves as an information source for individuals affected by blinding retinal degenerative diseases (such as retinitis pigmentosa, macular degeneration, and Usher syndrome), their families, and eye care professionals. Publishes *Fighting Blindness News* and *Macular Update*.

Glaucoma Foundation
33 Maiden Lane, 7th Floor
New York, NY 10038
(212) 504-1901 or (800) GLAUCOMA [452-8266]
FAX: (212) 504-1933
E-mail: glaucomafdn@mindspring.com
http://www.glaucomafoundation.org/info

Promotes and funds research into the causes of and potential cures for glaucoma. Provides free literature and referrals to the public, available through toll-free worldwide hotline.

Glaucoma Research Foundation
490 Post Street, Suite 830
San Francisco, CA 94102
(415) 986-3162 or (800) 826-6693
FAX: (415) 986-3763
E-mail: info@glaucoma.org
http://www.glaucoma.org

Works to protect the sight of individuals with glaucoma through research and education. Maintains a nationwide telephone glaucoma peer support network.

Lighthouse National Center for Vision and Aging
11 East 59th Street
New York, NY 10022
(212) 821-9200 or (800) 334-5497 or TDD (212) 821-9713
FAX: (212) 821-9705
http://www.lighthouse.org

Serves as a national clearinghouse for information on vision and aging and referrals to services.

Lions Eye Health Program
Lions Clubs International Foundation
300 22nd Street
Oak Brook, IL 60521-8842
(630) 571-5466
FAX: (630) 571-8890

Produces a quarterly newsletter on its eye health program.

Macular Degeneration, International
1968 West Ina Road, #106
Tucson, AZ 85741
(520) 797-2525 (FAX and telephone)

Serves persons with juvenile or age-related macular degeneration and supports research on finding the causes and treatments of macular degeneration.

National Association for Visually Handicapped
22 West 21st Street
New York, NY 10010
(212) 889-3141
FAX: (212) 727-2951

Provides services for the benefit of people with low vision, including information, large-print publications, counseling and peer-support sessions, and educational outreach programs for laypersons and professionals in the field of low vision.

National Eye Institute
National Institutes of Health
31 Center Drive, MSC 2510
Building 31, Room 6A32
Bethesda, MD 20892-2510
(301) 496-5248

Supports research on eye disease and the visual system. Provides free brochures on eye disorders. The National Eye Health Education Program provides public education packets on the four leading eye conditions associated with aging for use in conducting community education on preventing blindness.

National Federation of the Blind
1800 Johnson Street
Baltimore, MD 21230
(410) 659-9314
FAX: (410) 685-5653
http://www.nfb.org

Works to improve social and economic conditions of people who are blind or visually impaired and provides public education on related issues. Provides evaluations of present programs and assistance in establishing new ones. Has a public education program and affiliates in all states, the District of Columbia, and Puerto Rico. Publications include the *Braille Monitor.*

National Institute on Aging
National Institutes of Health
P.O. Box 8057
Gaithersburg, MD 20898-8057
(800) 222-2225 or TTD (800) 222-4225
http://www.nih.gov/nia

Provides funding for research on aging. Distributes *Age Pages* and other materials on a wide range of topics related to health and aging, including *Aging and Your Eyes.*

National Library Service for the Blind and Visually Handicapped
Library of Congress
1291 Taylor Street, N.W.
Washington, DC 20542
(800) 424-8567

Provides free library services to people with vision problems. Offers braille and large-print materials, recorded books, and other periodicals.

Prevent Blindness America
(formerly the National Society to Prevent Blindness)
500 East Remington Road
Schaumburg, IL 60173-5611
(800) 331-2020
FAX: (847) 843-8458
E-mail: preventblindness@compuserve.com
http://www.preventblindness.org

Conducts through a network of state affiliates a program of public and professional education, research, and industrial and community services to prevent blindness. Services include screening, vision testing, and dissemination of information on low-vision devices and clinics. Provides free pamphlets on specific diseases affecting the eyes. Offers Home Eye Test for Adults.

Vision Foundation
818 Mt. Auburn Street
Watertown, MA 02172
(617) 926-4232
FAX: (617) 926-1412

Publishes the Vision Resource List, which includes information on special products and services for people with visual impairments.

Sources of Products and Services

Low vision simulators or occluders—in the form of goggles that can be worn—are an excellent educational tool for helping students, professionals, service providers, volunteers, and family members understand functional vision limitations resulting from various eye conditions. The following organizations or individuals are suppliers or distributors of simulators.

Association for Education and Rehabilitation of the Blind and Visually Impaired (AER) Division 7 (Low Vision)
c/o Marshall Flax
354 West Main Street
Madison, WI 53703-3115
(608) 255-6178
FAX: (608) 255-3301
E-mail: Flax@Waisman.Wisc.Edu

Supplies a variety of simulators showing different degrees of various eye conditions, including age-related macular degeneration, retinitis pigmentosa, glaucoma, diabetic retinopathy, and cataracts.

AWARE (Associates for World Action Rehabilitation and Education)
P.O. Box 96
Mohegan Lake, NY 10547
(914) 528-0567
FAX: (914) 528-0567
E-mail: awareusa@aol.com

Publishes *New Independence for Older Persons with Vision Loss in Long-Term Care Facilities,* by M. Duffy and M. Toby-Beliveau, a package of training materials that includes low vision simulators.

The Lighthouse
11 East 59th Street
New York, NY 10022
(212) 821-9200 or (800) 334-5497 or TDD (212) 821-9713
FAX: (212) 821-9705
http://www.lighthouse.org

The VisualEyes Curriculum on vision rehabilitation for health and human service workers published by The Lighthouse contains vision simulators.

Dr. George Zimmerman
Program Coordinator
University of Pittsburgh
School of Education
Department of Instruction and Learning
4H01 Forbes Quadrangle
Pittsburgh, PA 15260
(412) 624-7254
FAX: (412) 648-7081
http://www:pitt.edu/~soeforum/sped_vis.html

Sells simulators.

FACT SHEET

What Is Low Vision?

Your vision is a complex sense made up of your ability to see contrasts and sharpness of detail and to evaluate the location of objects in the environment.

As you age your eyes change, but vision loss should not simply be accepted as a natural part of the aging process. In healthy aging eyes, changes in vision can be corrected by eyeglasses or contact lenses.

If you have been told by your eye care professional that your vision cannot be fully corrected by ordinary prescription lenses, medical treatment, or surgery, and you still have some usable vision, you have what is called "low vision."

Among older persons, low vision can result from specific eye conditions—such as macular degeneration, glaucoma, diabetic retinopathy and cataracts—or from a stroke.

If you have low vision, you may experience one or more of three types of vision problems. They are:

- *overall blurred vision*, which can be caused by cataracts, scars on the cornea or diabetic retinopathy
- *loss of central or center vision*, frequently caused by macular degeneration
- *loss of peripheral or side vision*, most commonly caused by glaucoma or stroke

There are ophthalmologists and optometrists with special training in low vision. Ask your eye care professional to refer you to a *low vision specialist* for a special kind of eye examination called a *low vision evaluation*. This specialist can determine the extent of your remaining vision and prescribe special optical devices that help you make the best use of the vision you have by magnifying the image you see, filtering light, or increasing the usable field of your vision.

Examples of low vision devices include:

- handheld or stand magnifiers and microscopic glasses for reading print or performing other close-up tasks
- frame-mounted or handheld pocket-sized telescopes for distance vision, such as reading a street sign or identifying the number of an approaching bus
- closed-circuit televisions for reading, which magnify and project printed materials onto a television screen
- high-intensity lamps or other nonoptical devices to enhance the use of residual vision for reading and other close-up tasks such as writing or sewing

You also may benefit from *vision-related rehabilitation services*, in which professionals can train you to use alternative methods to perform routine daily activities and to move about safely both indoors and outside your home. Ask your eye care professional to refer you to an agency that serves people who are visually impaired.

If you have low vision, you can continue to participate in activities you need to do and enjoy doing. Help is out there. See a low vision specialist!

Copyright © 1998, AFB Press

FACT SHEET

Tips for Making Print More Readable

Low vision often makes reading a difficult task. The conditions that cause low vision may affect the ability to read by

- reducing the amount of light that can enter the eye;
- blurring the image on the retina; or
- damaging the central portion of the retina (the macula) needed for fine vision.

The contrast of print against its background is affected by reduced light and blurring. Damage to the central retina interferes with the ability to see small print and to make the eye movements necessary for reading.

The following guidelines describe how to make print more legible for individuals with vision problems and for the general public as well.

Print Size

Use large-print type, preferably 18 point but a minimum of 16 point. Scalable fonts on the computer make this adjustment easy to do.

Font Type and Style

The goal in selecting type fonts or styles is to use easily recognizable characters, either standard roman or sans serif fonts. Avoid decorative fonts. **Use bold type because the thickness of the letters makes the print more legible.** Avoid using *italics* or ALL CAPITAL LETTERS. Both these forms of print make it more difficult to differentiate among letters.

Use of Color

Avoid using different-colored lettering for headings and emphasis; it is difficult to read for many people with low vision. When color is used, dark blues and greens are most effective.

Contrast

Contrast is one of the most critical factors in enhancing visual functioning, for printed materials as well as in environmental design. Text should be printed with the best possible contrast. For many older people, light lettering—either white or pale yellow—on a dark background, usually black, can be easier to read than black lettering on a white or pale yellow background.

Paper Quality

Avoid using glossy finish paper such as that typically used in magazines and some journals. Glossy pages create excess glare, which adds to the reading difficulty of people who have low vision.

Leading (Space Between Lines of Text)

The recommended spacing between lines of text is 1.5 spaces, rather than a single space. Many people who are visually impaired have difficulty finding the beginning of the next line when single spacing is used.

Spacing Between Letters

Text with letters spaced close together makes reading difficult for many people who are visually impaired, particularly those who have central visual field defects such as those accompanying macular degeneration. Spacing between letters should be wide.

(continued on following page)

Copyright © 1998, AFB Press

FACT SHEET

Making Print More Readable, continued

```
Mono-spaced fonts such as Courier,
which have an equal amount of
space allocated for each letter,
are easier to read.
```

Margins

Many low vision devices, such as stand magnifiers and closed-circuit televisions (CCTVs), are easiest to use on a flat surface. When materials are to be bound, printing them with an extra-wide binding margin (a minimum of 1 inch and preferably 1 1/2 inches if the material is thick) makes it easier to hold the material flat.

Copyright © 1998, AFB Press

FACT SHEET

Creating a Functional Environment for Older Individuals Who Are Visually Impaired

Making a private or public environment comfortable and functional for individuals who are blind or visually impaired should be part of environmental design for all older people, as such environments benefit older individuals in general.

Making facilities, programs, and activities safe and accessible for older participants who are blind or visually impaired need not necessarily require a great deal of time, energy, or money. It is a matter of knowing the basics and planning for easy access during the initial design of a facility and its programs.

The use of appropriate lighting, color contrast, and the reduction of glare are important factors of which architects and interior designers need to be aware, in order to create effective environmental design for older persons in general. Individuals working in the field of aging should take these vision factors into consideration when designing environments for older persons, particularly senior centers, retirement communities, assistive living environments, and nursing homes.

The suggestions presented here can be used to conduct an initial assessment of the environment. A vision rehabilitation professional can provide further assistance in assessing the environment and making recommendations for changes that will enhance safe and independent functioning and active participation.

The primary environmental elements to consider for older persons who are visually impaired, so that they may function independently in any environment, are the use of lighting and color contrast, placement of furniture, removal of obstacles and hazards in traffic areas, especially halls and stairways, and the placement and readability of signage.

The following are environmental adaptations or modifications that enhance functioning.

Lighting

- In recreation and reading areas, provide plenty of floor lamps and table lamps.
- Advise people who are visually impaired that light should always be aimed at the work they are doing, not at their eyes.
- Replace burned-out light bulbs.
- Place mirrors so that lighting does not reflect off them and create glare.
- For window coverings, use adjustable blinds, sheer curtains, or draperies, because they allow for the adjustment of natural light and the reduction of glare.
- Keep a few chairs near windows for reading or doing handicrafts in natural light.

Furniture

- Arrange furniture in small groupings so that people can converse easily.
- Make sure there is adequate lighting near furniture.
- When purchasing new furniture, select upholstery with texture whenever possible. Texture provides tactile clues for identification.

(continued on following page)

Copyright © 1998, AFB Press

FACT SHEET

Creating a Functional Environment, continued

- Use brightly colored accessories, such as vases and lamps, to create contrast and to make furniture easier to locate.
- Avoid upholstery and floor coverings that have patterns. Stripes and checks can create confusion for people who are visually impaired.

Elimination of Hazards

- Replace worn carpeting and floor covering.
- Tape down or remove area rugs.
- Remove electrical cords from pathways, or tape them down for safety.
- Do not wax floors; use nonskid, nonglare products to clean and polish floors.
- Keep chairs pushed in under desks and tables.
- Move large pieces of furniture out of the main traffic areas.
- If telephone booths protrude into main traffic areas, have them moved.

Use of Color Contrast

- Place objects against a contrasting background, for example, a dark table near a white wall or a black switchplate on a white wall.
- Install doorknobs that contrast in color with doors for easy location.
- Paint the woodwork of a door frame a contrasting color to make it easier to locate the door.
- Mark the edges of all steps and ramps with paint or tape of a highly contrasting color.

Hallways and Stairways

- In hallways, make sure that lighting is uniform throughout, using several light sources in long halls.
- Locate drinking fountains and fire extinguishers along one wall only throughout hallways, so that individuals who are visually impaired can trail along the other wall without encountering obstacles.
- Install grab bars wherever they may be needed.
- Light stairwells clearly.
- Make certain that stairway railings extend beyond the top and bottom steps.
- Mark landings in a highly contrasting color.

Signs

- Place all signs at eye level, and use large lettering that meets the specifications outlined in the Americans with Disabilities Act (ADA).
- Provide braille signage according to ADA specifications.
- Mark emergency exits clearly.
- When making signs by hand, use a heavy black felt-tip pen on a white, off-white, or light yellow, nonglossy background.

Telephones

- Provide some telephones with large-print keypads or dials.
- Provide telephone amplifiers, which increase the level of sound.

In-Home Modifications

The environmental elements described are

(continued on following page)

Copyright © 1998, AFB Press

FACT SHEET

Creating a Functional Environment, continued

also important for the older person with impaired vision to function independently and safely at home. Within the vision rehabilitation field, rehabilitation teachers—professionals who teach adaptive techniques for independent living—work with older persons who are visually impaired to make these environmental modifications within the home and in the workplace. If the rehabilitation teacher provides services in an older person's home, he or she can also assess that environment for safety and ease of functioning. Suggestions for modifications are usually easy to carry out because they typically involve few or low-cost changes that can be made by older people with a range of personal incomes.

For more information on easy, low-cost adaptations, see *Making Life More Livable*, by Irving Dickman (New York: American Foundation for the Blind, 1983).

Copyright © 1998, AFB Press

MODULE 3

The Psychosocial Aspects of Aging and Vision Loss: Impact on the Older Person, Family Members, and the Family Unit

This module provides an overview of the impact of vision loss on the older person and her or his family members within the context of the aging process. The aim is to prepare future service providers to:

- understand the nature of the life circumstances of an older person losing vision;
- know what services are available within the vision rehabilitation arena for older persons; and
- understand the responsibility of professionals to serve older visually impaired persons as mutual clients of the aging and blindness service delivery systems, and not just to refer them to the vision system.

This coordination of needs and appropriate services is essential to avoid fragmented service delivery and to provide for the individual's service needs.

Developing an understanding of the impact of vision loss on the older individual and family members begins with the context of aging in general and adds to that the specifics of vision loss. The view of the aging process presented here is that it is a time of positive experiences, while at the same time the realities of losses associated with growing older are acknowledged. The specific losses associated with visual impairment are placed within the context of other losses associated with the aging process; and the reactions to vision loss of both the older person and family members are explored. Finally, the process of adjustment and the need for vision-related rehabilitation services to enhance that adjustment are described.

Topic Outline

3.1 Theories of Aging

3.2 The Aging Process: Looking Forward to Later Years

3.3 Losses Associated with Aging

3.4 Perceived Loss and Real Loss

3.5 Losses Associated with Visual Impairment

3.6 Reactions to Vision Loss

　3.6.1 Reactions of Older Persons Experiencing Vision Loss

　3.6.2 Reactions of Family Members

3.7 Adjustment to Vision Loss

　3.7.1 Depression

　3.7.2 Reassessment and Reaffirmation

　3.7.3 Coping and Mobilizing

　3.7.4 The Role of Family Members

3.8 Vision Loss and Other Functional Limitations

3.9 The Need for Vision-Related Rehabilitation

3.1 Theories of Aging

Many theories of aging have been developed, particularly in the last four decades of the twentieth century. Some theories have focused

MODULE 3: THE PSYCHOSOCIAL ASPECTS OF AGING AND VISION LOSS

Learner Objectives

1. The student will be able to demonstrate a basic understanding of the psychosocial aspects of the aging process by describing both a positive view of aging and the losses associated with the aging process.
2. The student will be able to identify and describe the psychosocial issues associated with age-related vision loss for the older individual and family members.
3. The student will be able to describe the elements of the adjustment process and the individualized nature of adjusting to loss.
4. The student will be able to describe the impact of an older person's vision loss on his or her spouse and adult children.
5. The student will be able to describe the role of vision-related rehabilitation services, including support groups, for the older person who is newly visually impaired, as well as for family members.

on developmental tasks associated with the last stage of the life cycle. Others focus on the tasks associated with each stage of the life cycle (Erikson, 1963); therefore, an individual is characterized as moving successfully from one phase to another if he or she is able to accomplish the tasks associated with each phase.

In large measure, theories of aging are reflections of societal attitudes and perceptions about what is important and appropriate for each phase of the aging process and what the older individual's focus should be at each stage. Therefore, theories developed in the 1960s about the way to age successfully are considerably different from the views of gerontologists in the late 1990s.

These theories of aging have provided a framework in which to view and understand the impact of vision loss on the older person.

The current emphasis on productive aging or active aging is based on a broad definition of productive activity as well as an understanding of the older person's desire to continue to be productive.

Older people who lose their vision want to be, and are capable of being, self-sufficient, productive, contributing members of their families, their communities, and in many cases the work force. However, social attitudes frequently prevent the older person from reaching this potential.

3.2 The Aging Process: Looking Forward to Later Years

Older people typically look forward to some combination of the following life circumstances during their later years:

- being able to work as long as they wish
- enjoying planned retirement
- being productive in one or more arenas
- having positive and enriching relationships and maintaining a social network
- spending positive leisure time
- maintaining valued roles and identifying new positive roles
- functioning independently in their own homes
- experiencing a sense of interdependence (being both the provider and the recipient of care or assistance) within the family and social context
- making contributions to the family unit and the community
- traveling
- spending time with grandchildren
- identifying new opportunities for new learning
- discovering previously untapped skills and talents
- remaining in good physical and mental health

Older people who experience age-related vision loss want the same things and the same opportunities as other people their age; however, many of them perceive their desires to be beyond their grasp because of stereotypic thinking about blindness and disability in general that they learned in their youth.

Service providers in both the fields of aging and vision rehabilitation can help older consumers to realize that they can sustain or regain valued roles and activities. Access to vision-related rehabilitation services and participation in a support group with other newly visually impaired older persons can facilitate a person's adjustment to deteriorating vision.

3.3 Losses Associated with Aging

In spite of productive aging and the capacity for continued growth and development, the aging process is also associated with losses. The most typical losses include the following:

- loss of a spouse or significant other
- loss of siblings, neighbors, friends, and peers
- loss of geographic proximity to children and grandchildren
- loss of a social network
- loss of economic security
- loss of roles, particularly the work role
- loss of good health
- loss of aspects of physical functioning
- loss of physical and/or psychological mobility
- loss of self-worth or self-esteem
- loss of self-confidence and self-reliance
- loss of control over one's life
- loss of a sense of being whole

Any one of these losses can be traumatic, but when one loss is compounded by another, the individual's reaction is often intensified. New losses can evoke the painful experiences of prior losses.

3.4 Perceived Loss and Real Loss

It is initially difficult for the older person to distinguish between actual losses such as the loss of a loved one, a major role in life, or an aspect of physical functioning, and aspects of the loss that can be of short duration or overcome. It is important for professionals working with older people to help the individual make this differentiation.

Typically, when an older person experiences losses in functioning and psychological well-being, some of the feelings of loss, such as the feeling of loss of control, will dissipate over time if the person receives appropriate rehabilitation services. Older people can learn to adapt to a loss in physical functioning, and they can acquire new skills to restore and enhance psychosocial functioning disturbed by the loss.

3.5 Losses Associated with Visual Impairment

Losses associated with visual impairment are specific to vision loss, although they may also be characteristic of losses associated with other functional limitations. Father Thomas Carroll (1961) first outlined the losses associated with visual impairments. He divided them into six broad categories:

- losses of psychological security
- losses in basic skills
- losses in communication
- losses in appreciation
- losses concerning occupation and financial status
- resulting losses to the whole person

Some of the specific losses covered within these categories of primary losses are the following (Orr, 1991):

- loss of independence, or feeling the need to depend on someone else for everything
- loss of independent mobility, or feeling unable to move about familiar and unfamiliar environments
- loss of control over one's life, feeling unable to do anything or find anything in the environment; or complete disorientation
- loss of control over the physical environment, or feeling unable to locate anything ever again
- loss of the ability to drive a car
- loss of access to printed material; feeling cut off from the world; feeling less literate as a result of not having access to critical information contained in, for example, daily newspapers or mail related to eligibility requirements for benefits
- loss of privacy resulting from the need for assistance in many aspects of daily life, such as needing someone else to read one's personal mail
- loss of anonymity or obscurity in the world ("People will stare at me if I use a white cane").
- loss of written communication, or not being able to read letters and cards from loved ones or to write back
- loss of opportunity for nonverbal communication, or being unable to participate fully in group settings because of the inability to receive nonverbal feedback such as facial expressions and subtleties of body language
- loss of feelings of adequacy, self-esteem, and self-worth
- loss of roles and responsibilities, particularly the work role
- loss of opportunities for productive activity, particularly employment, volunteerism, participation in leisure activities, recreation, handicrafts, and hobbies

- loss of the feeling of social adequacy, or not feeling like an equal participant in a group activity or feeling unable to interact even with old friends
- loss of a sense of being whole, or feeling as though a piece of one's self is missing and the ability to function is gone

Understanding the losses associated with vision loss and the aging process enables family members and service providers to understand the issues that confront older persons when they experience vision loss, as well as the broad range of daily challenges and adjustments they face.

3.6 Reactions to Vision Loss

3.6.1 Reactions of Older Persons Experiencing Vision Loss

The older person experiencing age-related vision loss may undergo extensive emotional, cognitive, perceptual, and behavioral changes. Some of the reactions to vision loss that have been identified are similar to the five stages of the mourning process as outlined by Kübler-Ross (1969): denial, anger, bargaining, grief, and acceptance.

Tuttle (1984) identified typical reactions to vision loss and stages of adjustment pertaining specifically to vision loss, which also describe the harsh psychosocial process of coming to terms with any form of loss. They include the following stages:

- shock and denial
- anger and/or withdrawal
- succumbing and depression
- reassessment and reaffirmation
- coping and mobilization

These stages are discussed in more detail in the next section.

Loss of visual functioning evokes a similar set of reactions to those experienced with any loss—whether the loss of a loved one, the loss of a limb, or the loss of a degree of functioning. Both the mourning process and the adjustment process occur along a continuum, from pushing the reality away at one end, to allowing the reality to take hold and experiencing the pain, to finally taking steps toward recovery. The older individual's reactions to vision loss may include any or all of the following, in any combination and any order or sequence.

- *Shock or denial of the vision loss.* The older person may feel numb when first informed about his/her eye condition. The numbness may then turn into denial that he or she has a vision problem. The older person may continue to carry out various activities independently in spite of serious difficulty and safety risks to him- or herself and others—for example, crossing streets without assistance, continuing to cook when unable to regulate the stove flame or see where to position a pot, or continuing to drive when no longer able to see clearly. The older person may also manifest denial by going from doctor to doctor looking for a more encouraging diagnosis or medical treatment, even when told that there is no medical intervention available to restore vision.
- *Anger at living longer, but not necessarily "better."* Older people may express anger and frustration at their situation, and they may direct their anger at those closest to them, typically family members.
- *Feelings of deterioration and vulnerability.* Older people may experience a sense that they are physically falling apart and that as they age, one loss in functioning will lead to another in an inevitable downward spiral.
- *Despair and hopelessness.* Vision loss can be an isolating experience; both the physical and psychological isolation can lead to feelings of hopelessness and despair about the present and perceived lack of future. Feelings of deep despair make it difficult for the older person to take steps toward seeking and accepting help, perpetuating a vicious cycle.
- *Social isolation as a result of psychological withdrawal.* Older people may withdraw from previously valued social activities and friends because of feelings of inadequacy or because they can no longer travel. In addition, people in their social networks may decrease their involvement with the newly visually impaired individuals because of their own discomfort and fear of vision loss. Isolation is one of the most common experiences and difficulties associated with age-related vision loss. Withdrawal may lead to a loss of control over their life. They may also begin to perceive themselves as homebound and in need of more help than they actually require.
- *Fear.* Older people may fear other impending losses of functioning or catastrophic illness. Another common fear is the threat of nursing home placement, with the associated loss of autonomy and depletion of life savings.
- *Grief and mourning.* Experiencing grief, although painful and difficult, is a positive sign of the individual's movement through the

adjustment process. The grieving process may be exhibited in crying and sobbing, along with a recognition of loss, or talking repeatedly about the way things used to be before the vision loss. The individual mourns for the lost vision and the activities it permitted in the same way one mourns the loss of a loved one.

Support and encouragement, good advice, and access to information can help the older individual and family members take steps toward adjustment. (See Modules 5 and 6 and the Resources at the end of this module for information on support groups and other supportive services. See the fact sheets at the end of this module and Module 2 for consumer information on aging and vision loss.)

3.6.2 Reactions of Family Members

People who are extremely close to an older person, especially adult children and spouses, may find themselves experiencing some of the following fears and feelings in response to the older person's experience with age-related vision loss.

- *Fear that the older person will be unable to function independently.* Family members frequently worry that their visually impaired relative will not be able to continue to live at home, will have to move in with adult children, or will need 24-hour in-home long-term care or nursing home placement.
- *Fears concerning the older family member's safety, particularly when the older family member wants to continue to do things independently.*
- *The desire to reverse roles and do everything for the older family member.* Adult children frequently think it is now their turn to take care of the parent as the parent took care of them.
- *Feelings of having lost a parent as someone to turn to for advice or comfort as they did in the past.*
- *Feelings of being overwhelmed or burdened with responsibilities or worries.*
- *Feelings of helplessness.* Family members may not know where to turn for help.
- *Uncertainty about when to help and when to step back.*
- *Uncertainty about whether to talk about the loss with the older individual.* Family members may be unsure about whether to initiate discussion or wait for the older person to begin to express feelings or concerns.

Family members—spouses and adult children in particular—experience their own grief and need to go through an individual mourning process. They may be in constant conflict, trying to resolve their own feelings while at the same time having to deal with the reactions of the individual who has experienced the vision loss.

3.7 Adjustment to Vision Loss

No one adjusts to change, to loss, or to impairment in a vacuum. Adjustment occurs within the familial and social context. An individual's ability to adjust and the rate of adjustment depend on many factors, including individual coping strategies established during the life cycle and the involvement and reactions of significant others.

Several factors are critical to keep in mind in trying to understand an individual's reaction to vision loss and progress through the stages of adjustment:

- Adjustment to any change, even a positive change, is a process.
- Adjustment occurs in incremental steps and stages, which build on each other to restore physical and psychological well-being.
- Although there are basic stages to adjusting to vision loss as to any other loss, the stages are not necessarily sequential.
- One phase need not be completed before another phase begins.
- A phase is not necessarily completed because the older individual moves to another phase.
- The older person experiencing vision loss may shift back and forth among phases before achieving a level of adjustment.

The older person's pattern of adjustment is influenced by internal and external factors. Internal factors include the following:

- The individual's current state of physical well-being
- the individual's typical or patterned responses to change, stress, or crisis
- the presence or absence of other health conditions
- religious and cultural beliefs

External factors include the following:

- the presence or absence of supportive loved ones
- perceptions and attitudes about disability in general and about vision loss in particular (see Module 5)
- knowing another older person who is visually impaired and whether or not that individual is in a state of despair, is surviving,

or is thriving (see Module 6 for a discussion of peer support groups and peers as instructors, counselors, and mentors)
- awareness of essential vision-related services, including low vision services and vision rehabilitation services, and how to gain access to such services (see Modules 4 and 5 for discussions of vision-related services and how to obtain access to them)

These factors indicate how complex and confusing the adjustment process can be for the older individual and family members, and why it takes considerable time for many individuals.

3.7.1 Depression

The experience of sadness and depression is normal and necessary to the adjustment process. Depression may occur or recur at any time along the adjustment continuum.

3.7.2 Reassessment and Reaffirmation

The reassessment and reaffirmation stage of adjustment (Tuttle, 1984) begins when the individual moves through the earlier phases and is characterized by the following psychological process. The older person

- identifies his or her own strengths and weaknesses,
- affirms his or her individual personal belief systems,
- recognizes that there can be a future, and
- starts to plan for that future.

3.7.3 Coping and Mobilizing

In general, individuals will try to learn techniques to keep themselves independent to the extent they wish to be or care to be. Some techniques are adaptive and others are maladaptive, but both adaptive and maladaptive strategies are ways of coping with difficult situations. In the coping and mobilizing phase of adjustment (Tuttle, 1984), the individual develops strategies to cope with vision loss.

Adaptive responses and techniques use inner resources and previously developed coping strategies, as well as external resources, to adjust to vision loss. Adaptive responses can be characterized as follows:

- maintaining typical social behavioral patterns
- continuing to try to carry out activities of daily living (ADLs), including bathing, dressing, using the toilet, grooming, eating, and

transferring from bed to a chair, as well as instrumental activities of daily living (IADLs), including preparing meals, feeding, housekeeping, doing the laundry, taking medication, managing money, walking outside, grocery shopping, and using public transit

Maladaptive responses include dependent and inactive forms of behaviors beyond those associated with loss in general or with vision loss specifically. An unwillingness to accept assistance or to take advantage of services, including vision-related rehabilitation services, can be a maladaptive response.

Maladaptive responses also include giving up valued behaviors and activities, such as going outside the home, attending religious services, attending a senior center, doing volunteer work, participating in social and recreational activities, or attending to personal appearance and housekeeping.

3.7.4 The Role of Family Members

The role of family members is critical to the adjustment process. Their reactions and patterns of interaction can have a tremendous impact on the older individual. Family members can play a facilitating or inhibiting role in how the older person deals with the loss of vision.

Because individual family members each have their own set of reactions and adjustment process, key family members frequently are not at similar stages in the adjustment process. This complicates the adjustment process within the family unit.

Supportive family members can make a major difference in an individual's adjustment, primarily because they can be emotionally available for the older family member as she or he moves through the fear, denial, and anger and becomes ready to accept services and to make the adaptations needed to carry out basic activities and to become involved in life again. (See the fact sheet on "When an Older Person Experiences Vision Loss: Tips for Family Members" at the end of this module.)

3.8 Vision Loss and Other Functional Limitations

The combination of vision loss with other health or physical conditions that impair mobility, such as arthritis, can seriously limit mobility to the extent that the older person experiences a shrinking physical environment.

Similarly, when an older individual experiences vision loss along with other sensory impairments, particularly hearing loss, it intensifies the social impact, shrinking the psychosocial environment.

Vision loss has an even greater impact when it occurs together with chronic or acute physical health problems, or in combination with forms of dementia, such as Alzheimer's disease.

The more service providers know about the life circumstances associated with loss of vision as part of the aging process and other concomitant losses, the more successful their interventions can be.

3.9 The Need for Vision-Related Rehabilitation

The most important message for the older person experiencing vision loss is that help is available. Age-related eye conditions may cause loss of vision that cannot be restored medically or surgically, but there are services and devices (described in Module 4) that can enable the older individual to make the best use of remaining vision. Learning adaptive techniques to carry out routine tasks is crucial; the adjustment is often difficult, but access to services and support can make a major difference in the individual's quality of life.

Independent living services for older persons who are blind or severely visually impaired can enhance their quality of life, promote independence, and reduce dependence on relatives and ongoing supportive services. The loss of the ability to carry out basic life skills such as cooking, handling household chores, using the telephone, and identifying money may result in unnecessary and costly institutionalization. It is this outcome that independent living services for older persons who are blind or visually impaired were designed to avoid.

Testifying before the U.S. House of Representatives Select Committee on Aging at the 1985 hearing on the federally funded Independent Living Services for Older Individuals Who Are Blind program (see Module 4), a retired physician who had lost her sight and was placed in a nursing home spoke the following words:

> My doctor didn't know what else to do with me. My doctor never made mention of a program available to rehabilitate the visually impaired or any of the aids and devices currently on the market which enable the blind to carry out daily living tasks. If he had, I

could have been spared the five months of frustration, anger, and depersonalization I experienced while in the nursing home. (cited in Rogers, 1997)

At last a friend put her in touch with a rehabilitation agency that served people who are blind or visually impaired, and she was trained in independent living skills. The result, she stated, was that

> special training has given me back my freedom and my independence. I am once again a responsible adult making my own decisions and living my own life. Losing one's sight is not the end of one's existence. You simply need to relearn how to do basic tasks with a few adaptations. I am grateful to be in my own home again. Yet, I wonder how many other elderly people with a vision loss are trapped within the walls of a nursing home when they too could be in their own home living a full and independent life.

Professionals with specialized training in blindness and visual impairment can play a major role in enabling people who are older and blind or visually impaired to maximize their capacity for independent living.

Many older individuals who experience age-related vision loss have no conception of vision rehabilitation services, of how to gain access to these services, or of their potential to live more independently. They need education about these possibilities, and they also need help to overcome any stereotypic views they may hold about blindness and aging.

Some older individuals may reject assistance for the following key reasons:

- fear of admitting that they have a vision problem and that they need assistance
- loss of self-esteem or self-confidence or feelings of uselessness and worthlessness
- anger or depression

Moreover, each individual, as well as each family member, deals with the impact of vision loss differently. Each individual varies in the amount of time he or she needs to adjust to the situation and be ready to move to the next step of seeking and accepting vision-related services. Frequently, the older individual and key family members are not at the same stages of readiness to move forward.

This phenomenon can affect the older individual's progress in learning and utilizing new skills for independent living.

For example, an older person may be ready to inquire about the kinds of help available, but her or his adult child may still want to do everything for the parent, believing this to be best for the parent. The reverse may also occur. An adult child may realize how time-consuming and maladaptive it is to do everything for the parent and may be ready to seek assistance from outside the family, but the parent may still be too depressed to accept outside services and want to have no part of the adult child's plan.

By recognizing the array of reactions, feelings, and stages of adjustment within the family, a trained rehabilitation professional or a professional outside the vision field can assist the older individual, and family members as well, with the adjustment process.

Older people experiencing vision loss who receive special independent living services have the enhanced opportunity to regain their self-esteem, be able to take care of their personal and daily living needs, move about the home, walk to the mailbox, travel to the local supermarket, reach a senior center and other destinations safely, and feel more confident being involved in the community again. These are small tasks that are taken for granted until they can no longer be performed because of a vision problem (Rogers, 1997).

References

Carroll, T. J. (1961). *Blindness: What it is, what it does, and how to live with it.* Boston: Little, Brown.

Erikson, E. (1963). *Childhood and society.* New York: W. W. Norton.

Kübler-Ross, E. (1969). *On death and dying.* New York: Macmillan.

Orr, A. L. (1991). The psychosocial aspects of aging and vision loss. *Journal of Gerontological Social Work, 17*(3–4), 1–14.

Rogers, P. (1997). *Impact of specialized independent living programs for older people experiencing vision loss.* In J. Scott, L. Lidoff, & A. L. Orr (Eds.), *Advocacy tools.* New York: American Foundation for the Blind, National Aging and Vision Network.

Tuttle, D. (1984). *Self-esteem and adjusting with blindness.* Springfield, IL: Charles C Thomas.

RECOMMENDED TEACHING METHODS

Small-Group Brainstorming

Organize students into small groups of four or five students, to make a list of the typical losses associated with the aging process. Have each group report, and create a composite list for the class.

Ask the small groups to brainstorm about the losses specifically associated with vision loss among older persons, then report back to the large group. Create an exhaustive list from the group reports.

Lecture

Give an overview of the developmental tasks associated with the aging process in dealing with loss in general and the impact of vision loss in particular. Integrate the ideas gathered during the small-group brainstorming sessions.

Videotapes

Show one or more of the videotapes listed in the Resources section. After viewing each film, the following questions can be used to explore the issues raised:

- What was the primary message in the film?
- Which character was most effective in delivering the message?
- With whom did you identify in the film?

Role Play

Organize students into small groups to develop a case scenario of a family in which an older woman has gradually lost some of her vision. The family includes her spouse, adult son and daughter, and their spouses. Ask each group to develop the characters, focusing on their reactions and feelings associated with the older person's vision loss. Then have each group of students role play the scenario they have developed.

Give students a minimum of 20 minutes to develop the scenario and 10 to 15 minutes for each role play. Have students in the observing groups analyze the family dynamics and discuss whether they are functional or dysfunctional.

Large-Group Discussion

Referring students to the role-playing scenarios, ask them to analyze family members' expressions of feelings and reactions to the older visually impaired woman. Discuss where each family member is in the adjustment process.

Guest Speakers

Invite a vision rehabilitation professional from a local agency to discuss the vision-related rehabilitation services available to older individuals, including support groups for older people and family members.

Invite someone from a support group in the area to talk about the role of the group in adjusting to and coping with late-life vision loss.

Fact Sheets

The fact sheets included in this module may be useful for distribution to students. They have been written with the older consumer and family members in mind. They also can be used by students for projects, such as developing a public education campaign on age-related vision loss.

RESOURCES

Recommended Readings

Burack-Weiss, A. (1991). In their own words. In N. D. Weber (Ed.), *Vision and aging: Issues in social work practice*. New York: Haworth Press.

Burack-Weiss, A. (1993). Psychosocial aspects of aging and vision loss. In E. E. Faye & C. Stuen (Eds.), *The aging eye and low vision: A study guide for physicians* (pp. 15–23). New York: The Lighthouse National Center for Vision and Aging.

Crews, J. E., & Frey, W. D. (1993). Family concerns and older people who are blind. *Journal of Visual Impairment & Blindness, 87,* 6–11.

Flax, M. E., Golembiewski, D. J., & McCaulley, B. L. (1993). *Coping with vision loss.* San Diego: Singular Publishing Group.

Orr, A. L. (1991). The psychosocial aspects of aging and vision. In N. D. Weber (Ed.), *Vision and aging: Issues in social work practice* (pp. 1–14). New York: Haworth Press.

Orr, A. L. (1994). Understanding the impact of vision loss on the older person. In S. E. Boone, D. Watson, & M. Bagley (Eds.), *The challenge to independence: Vision and hearing loss among older adults,* (pp. 127–138). Little Rock: University of Arkansas Rehabilitation Research and Training Center.

Ringgold, N. (1991). *Out of the corner of my eye.* New York: American Foundation for the Blind.

Van Zandt, P. L., Van Zandt, S. L., & Wang, A. (1994). The role of support groups in the adjustment to visual impairment in old age. *Journal of Visual Impairment & Blindness, 88,* 244–252.

Further Reading

Dodds, A., Ferguson, E., Ng, L., Flannigan, H., Hawes, G., & Yates, L. (1994). The concept of adjustment: A structural model. *Journal of Visual Impairment & Blindness, 88*(6), 487–497.

Nixon, H. L (1994). Looking sociologically at a family coping with visual impairment. *Journal of Visual Impairment & Blindness, 88*(4), 329–337.

Jackson, R., & Lawson, G. (1995). Family environment and psychological distress in persons who are visually impaired. *Journal of Visual Impairment & Blindness, 89*(2), 157–160.

Stuen, C. (1994). Self-help/mutual aid support groups for visually impaired older adults. In S. E. Boone, D. Watson, & M. Bagley (Eds.), *The challenge to independence: Understanding vision and hearing loss in older adults* (pp. 139–146). Little Rock: University of Arkansas Rehabilitation Research and Training Center.

Videotapes

Aging and vision: Declarations of independence. (1984). New York: American Foundation for the Blind.

A personal look at five older people who have coped successfully with visual impairment and continue to lead active, satisfying lives. Their stories are not only inspirational but also provide practical, down-to-earth suggestions for adapting to vision loss later in life.

Look out for Annie. (1987). New York: The Lighthouse.
A review of the issues that arise when an older person loses vision in later life. It includes issues related to the mother-daughter relationship and to participation in a senior center. The video is especially effective for community education, in-service training, and support groups for older persons and their family members. Includes a discussion guide.

Blindness: A family matter. (1986). New York: American Foundation for the Blind.
A frank exploration of the effects of an individual's visual impairment on other members of the family and how these family members can play a positive role in the vision rehabilitation process. The characters are not older persons; however, the family relationships and interpersonal dynamics are relevant. Features interviews with three families whose success stories provide advice and encouragement, as well as interviews with newly blind adults who are currently involved in a vision-related rehabilitation program.

Other Materials

A directory of self-help mutual aid support groups for older people with impaired vision. (1994). New York: The Lighthouse.
A directory containing state-by-state listings of over 670 support groups, plus self-help clearinghouses, state agencies for the blind and visually impaired, private vision rehabilitation agencies that work with older people, national resource organizations, and a bibliography of books and articles on organizing and facilitating support groups.

Sharing solutions. New York: The Lighthouse.
Newsletter in which older people across the country who are experiencing vision loss share information and experiences.

FACT SHEET

When an Older Person Experiences Vision Loss: Tips for Family Members

If you are the spouse, adult child, or another close relative of an older person with vision loss, you are not alone. There are already approximately 5 million older Americans experiencing vision loss severe enough to interfere with their ability to function independently.

In the United States, more than 80 percent of the supportive assistance and care needed by older people who are limited in their ability to function independently is provided by family caregivers. Family members and significant others are a powerful source of support for the older person who is experiencing vision loss.

When a family member experiences deteriorating vision, the rest of the family feels the emotional impact. They worry that their relative may become depressed, isolated, and dependent. But with the right services and training, the older person can continue to be independent and productive. You can help in the following ways.

Encourage Eye Examinations

- Make sure your relative is examined by an eye care professional—an ophthalmologist or an optometrist.
- Be certain, too, that your relative is evaluated by a low vision specialist—usually an optometrist with a specialization in low vision. The low vision specialist can help your older relative make the best use of remaining vision by prescribing low vision devices such as handheld magnifiers, high-intensity lighting, and others.

Know About Vision-Related Rehabilitation Services

- Get to know about vision-related rehabilitation services provided by state and private agencies serving blind and visually impaired persons. These include independent living skills training—learning adaptive techniques for carrying out activities of daily living—and orientation and mobility training—learning how to orient oneself to familiar and unfamiliar environments and how to move about within them, including travel with the use of a long white cane.
- Find out how to obtain these rehabilitation services by contacting your state agency serving blind and visually impaired people or a local private agency serving older persons who are visually impaired.

Support Your Relative During Vision Rehabilitation

- When you find out about the rehabilitation services in your community, explain them to your family member. Encourage your relative to participate, but leave the decision up to him or her.
- Get involved in the independent living skills training. Learn as many of the adaptive techniques as you can. That way you can offer encouragement to your relative and reinforce the new skills.
- Encourage your relative to be independent at home and in the community. It can help

(continued on following page)

Copyright © 1998, AFB Press

FACT SHEET

Tips for Family Members, continued

to make adaptations within the home, such as rearranging furniture for greater ease of movement, improving lighting, and using contrasting colors for greater visibility.

Make the Adjustment Process a Family Matter

- Encourage open communication among family members about the impact of vision loss on individual family members.
- Support your visually impaired family member's interest and ability to continue or resume important activities and tasks.
- Create opportunities for interdependence among members of the family. Remember that your visually impaired relative can be both a recipient and a provider of assistance within the family across generations.
- Find out from a local agency serving older persons who are blind or visually impaired if there are support groups for people who are newly visually impaired. Also inquire about family caregiver support groups. If such groups don't exist, think about starting one!

Remember, your family member can still be a productive and contributing member of your family and your community. You can help your relative look toward a future of independence, self-esteem, and self-confidence.

Copyright © 1998, AFB Press

FACT SHEET

Maintaining Your Independence After Vision Loss

If you experience vision loss, vision-related rehabilitation services and devices can help you continue to live in your own home and community. The place to start is with your eye care professional.

An ophthalmologist diagnoses and treats eye conditions and diseases, in some cases prescribing medications or surgery to improve or prevent the worsening of vision-related conditions. An optometrist diagnoses eye conditions and can prescribe corrective lenses. If the vision loss cannot be completely corrected and interferes with your everyday living, then it is time to consider vision-related rehabilitation services to help maintain or restore independent living skills. Such rehabilitation can help you regain your self-sufficiency and quality of life.

What Are Vision-Related Rehabilitation Services?

Vision-related rehabilitation services can restore functioning after vision loss, just as physical therapy restores function after a person loses the use of a limb. Vision-related rehabilitation services include the following:

1. low vision examinations and devices (such as handheld magnifiers, high-intensity lamps, and other optical and nonoptical aids) designed to help you make the best use of remaining vision
2. individual counseling to help in the adjustment to vision loss
3. support groups that provide the opportunity to talk with others about similar problems and ways to cope
4. Training in adaptive techniques to restore your skills in the following areas:

   - home and personal management, including meal preparation, personal care techniques, managing money, and labeling medications
   - communication, including the use of readers, tape recorders, braille, large print, computers with synthetic screen and screen magnification, writing guides, telephones, and timepieces
   - independent movement and travel, including orienting yourself in familiar and unfamiliar environments, asking for assistance from others when appropriate, and moving about using a long white cane or other devices

These services can make a big difference in the lives of older persons and their family members.

Who Provides Vision-Related Rehabilitation?

Services are provided by specially trained vision rehabilitation professionals, such as:

- orientation and mobility specialists
- rehabilitation teachers
- rehabilitation technology specialists
- low vision instructors
- vision rehabilitation therapists

Where Can You Find These Services?

Many communities have private agencies

(continued on following page)

Copyright © 1998, AFB Press

FACT SHEET

Maintaining Your Independence, continued

that serve people who are blind or visually impaired. Don't be put off by the word "blind" in an agency's name, because most agencies assist people with varying degrees of vision loss.

Some agencies have fees for services; others do not. Consult your local telephone directory, or call the American Foundation for the Blind for a referral at 1-800-232-5463.

Persons age 55 or older who are experiencing vision loss that interferes with daily living may be able to benefit from a federally funded program called Independent Living Services for Older Individuals Who Are Blind (Title VII, Chapter 2 of the Rehabilitation Act). Services are available at no charge to people age 55 and older who have severe visual impairments. You do not need to be totally blind to qualify. Program requirements vary from state to state. Contact the state's rehabilitation agency for information.

Some rehabilitation services may be offered by low vision care clinics, but be aware that Medicare and other health insurance policies do not usually cover these services. Ask your ophthalmologist or optometrist for further information.

Copyright © 1998, AFB Press

MODULE 4

Community-Based Services for Older Persons Who Are Blind or Visually Impaired

Older persons who experience vision loss can continue to be active, productive, and contributing members of their families and communities with the help of vision-related rehabilitation services. Many older persons and their family members are still not aware of the vision rehabilitation services available to them. In addition, many may resist seeking help from an agency that has the word "blind" in its name because they have difficulty identifying themselves as blind or severely visually impaired. As many as five to seven years may pass from the onset of vision loss until many older people seek assistance and get the help they need to function independently.

Topic Outline

4.1 Legislation and Funding for Vision-Related Rehabilitation Services

   4.1.1 The Rehabilitation Act of 1973 and Its Amendments

   4.1.2 Funding for the Chapter 2 Independent Living Program

**MODULE 4:
COMMUNITY-BASED SERVICES
FOR OLDER PERSONS
WHO ARE BLIND
OR VISUALLY IMPAIRED**

    4.1.3 Services Provided by the Independent Living Program

    4.1.4 Outcomes of Chapter 2 Services

4.2 The Vision-Related Rehabilitation Service Delivery System

    4.2.1 Service Delivery Structure

    4.2.2 Specialized Services for Older Individuals

4.3 Specialized Vision-Related Rehabilitation Professionals

    4.3.1 Andragogy: Principles of Adult Learning

    4.3.2 Rehabilitation Teaching

    4.3.3 Assessment, Planning, and Evaluation

    4.3.4 Orientation and Mobility

    4.3.5 Low Vision Services

Learner Objectives

1. The student will be able to identify and describe the array of vision-related services available to ameliorate the impact of age-related vision loss.

2. The student will be able to identify and describe the specialized vision rehabilitation professionals and the services they provide.

3. The student will be able to list and describe the significance of rehabilitation legislation, its history, and current legislative issues.

4. The student will be able to describe the background and current status of the Title VII, Chapter 2 Independent Living Services for Older Individuals Who Are Blind program and the legislative advocacy needed to preserve this program.

5. The student will be able to describe the significance of specialized vision-related rehabilitation services and the funding needed to meet the growth in the population of older persons experiencing age-related vision loss.

6. The student will be able to describe the key role that he or she can play as a professional in the aging network or related field in facilitating access to vision-related rehabilitation services for older individuals.

4.4 Rehabilitation Teaching Methods and Learning Environments
  4.4.1 Home-Based Model
  4.4.2 Agency-Based Model
  4.4.3 Combined Model

4.1 Legislation and Funding for Vision-Related Rehabilitation Services

4.1.1 The Rehabilitation Act of 1973 and Its Amendments

The Rehabilitation Act of 1973 was landmark legislation for individuals with a broad range of disabilities. This legislation reflected a major commitment on the part of Congress to the rehabilitation of individuals with disabilities to prepare them to return to work.

The 1978 amendments to this act were noteworthy in that they established an independent living program for individuals with disabilities whose rehabilitation goal was independent living, rather than remunerative employment. Title VII, the section of the act created by these amendments, authorized funds for independent living services. Parts A and B (now referred to as Chapter 1) provide funds for independent living services for all individuals with disabilities, as well as for independent living centers. Part C (now called Chapter 2) authorized grants to state vocational rehabilitation agencies to serve older individuals who are blind or severely visually impaired by providing training in independent living skills.

For purposes of this program, "older individual who is blind" was defined as "an individual age 55 or older whose severe visual impairment makes competitive employment extremely difficult to attain but for whom independent living goals are feasible." Title VII, Chapter 2 put the rehabilitation needs of older people on the public policy agenda for the first time. (Basic information about the program is summarized in the fact sheet on the Independent Living Services for Older Individuals Who Are Blind program at the end of this module.)

It is important to understand some of the history behind the Title VII, Chapter 2 program because of the extensive efforts required to bring this program to fruition. It was only after considerable legislative advocacy, including public hearings featuring testimony about the needs of the growing population of older people experiencing

MODULE 4: COMMUNITY-BASED SERVICES FOR OLDER PERSONS WHO ARE BLIND OR VISUALLY IMPAIRED

vision loss, the lack of services to this group, and the lack of funds to provide these services, that a separate part of Title VII was designated specifically for older Americans who were blind or severely visually impaired. Extensive details about Chapter 2 are provided here because of its significance to the vision rehabilitation field and to the field of aging as well.

4.1.2 Funding for the Chapter 2 Independent Living Program

All Rehabilitation Act funds are administrated at the federal level by the Rehabilitation Services Administration (RSA), which is part of the U.S. Department of Education, Office of Special Education and Rehabilitation Services. Funds are filtered down to state rehabilitation agencies. (More details about the structure of the service delivery system are provided in Module 5.)

Although the 1978 reauthorization of the Rehabilitation Act established the independent living program, the program did not receive legislative priority, and funds were not allocated for what was then Title VII, Part C until 1986. With the first appropriation in 1986, funds were awarded on a discretionary basis, requiring states to compete for available dollars. Twenty-five grants of approximately $200,000 each were awarded to the state rehabilitation agencies that submitted the best proposals.

This discretionary grant procedure created a number of problems. In states that did not receive these funds, and in which the state agency was the only agency serving blind and visually impaired persons, older visually impaired persons received few or no vision-related rehabilitation services.

Moreover, states funded in one round of funding were not guaranteed funding in the next round. Also, because states were competing for the same pool of limited funds, state agency personnel did not feel free to share information about the types of services they were developing with other state agencies. As a result, programs did not benefit from the sharing that later became possible, and states worked in isolation, duplicating their efforts rather than benefiting from each others' experience and acquired expertise.

From the inception of the independent living program, advocates for the older visually impaired population called for a legislative change from this discretionary grant program to a formula grant mechanism. Formula funding would fund each state at the same specified level, but states with a larger elderly population would receive an additional amount based on the number of individuals eligible for services. Thus, each state would have an equitable distribution of funds, and the competition for funds among the states at each round of funding would be eliminated.

The 1992 reauthorization of the Rehabilitation Act altered the funding mechanism of Title VII, Chapter 2 to a formula grant, to be implemented upon allocation of $13 million to the program, which was then allocated only $8.1 million. Thus, once the annual appropriation reaches $13 million, the program will convert to a formula grant program, with an allocation assured to every state.

In the meantime, consideration was given at the federal level to dividing the allocation among all 50 states so that each state would have some portion of the limited funds available to serve visually impaired older persons. To eliminate the possibility of a state losing or gaining funding from funding cycle to funding cycle, an agreement was made between RSA and the National Council of State Agencies for the Blind (NCSAB) to fund a larger number of Chapter 2 programs, each at a reduced rate, in order to create a more equitable situation among states. RSA also lengthened the funding cycle from three to five years, increasing the stability within each state program.

For the first time in 1995, all viable applications for Chapter 2 funds were funded, 48 states in all. For fiscal years 1995 and 1996, approximately $8.9 million was appropriated each year. This appropriation allowed for state grants ranging from $140,000 to $180,000. In FY 1996, every state received a grant for the first time.

In 1997, when the appropriation was $9.9 million, advocates for Chapter 2 recommended that Chapter 2 funds for 1998 be increased to $52 million to meet the needs of all older individuals throughout the country who are blind or visually impaired. The $52 million figure was established by NCSAB to represent the amount needed to provide a truly equitable level of funds across the country. Although it was obvious that Congress would not increase the allocation by such a dramatic amount, advocates for the program joined the effort to demonstrate a unified voice and to educate legislators about the real needs of this burgeoning population.

The National Aging and Vision Network, a national advocacy group convened by specialists in aging at the American Foundation

MODULE 4:
COMMUNITY-BASED SERVICES
FOR OLDER PERSONS
WHO ARE BLIND
OR VISUALLY IMPAIRED

for the Blind, has led a national advocacy campaign to preserve the integrity of Chapter 2 as well as to increase its funding. The very existence of the program has been challenged by those who argue that Title VII, Chapter 1 of the Rehabilitation Act—which provides independent living services for individuals with all types of disabilities—should absorb the Chapter 2 program. Older individuals who are blind or visually impaired would then be served by independent living centers along with individuals with all other types of disabilities, rather than receiving specialized vision-related rehabilitation services targeted to that population. This issue reemerges each time the Rehabilitation Act is up for reauthorization. (For a further discussion of the threats to specialized vision-related services, see Module 6.)

Title VII, Chapter 2 has been the only consistent source to provide funding for vision-related rehabilitation services for older individuals. Medicare, Medicaid, and private insurance traditionally have not covered vision-related rehabilitation services or adaptive devices.

The vision field has been working toward positioning vision-related rehabilitation services and the field's specialized personnel for such third-party reimbursement, however, and some agencies have begun to develop mechanisms to obtain third-party reimbursement (see Module 6). As the population requiring services grows, increasing and diversifying funding streams to keep pace with the need for services are critical concerns.

4.1.3 Services Provided by the Independent Living Program

A wide variety of services may be provided through the Title VII, Chapter 2 program, such as independent living skills training, orientation and mobility (O&M) training, low vision services, the provision of adaptive devices (optical and nonoptical as funds permit), individual and family counseling, and community integration (including outreach and information and referral).

Each state utilizes Chapter 2 funds to design its own program model to meet the specific needs of its population of older visually impaired individuals.

The core services outlined under Title VII, Chapter 2—and therefore the services most frequently provided—are the following:

- training for activities of daily living

- the provision of adaptive devices such as those used for cooking safely, large-print or braille clocks and watches, and closed-circuit televisions, as funds permit
- O&M training
- training in communication skills and the use of communication devices
- low vision services
- family and peer counseling
- community integration, including outreach and information and referral

An annual analysis of the program's achievements (Herndon, 1993; Moore & Stephens, 1995; Stephens, 1994, 1996) describes the specific services provided within the core categories. Following are some examples to provide an understanding of the scope of the Chapter 2 program.

- Activities of daily living
    - cooking classes, including microwave cooking
    - two-week residential school programs for independent living skills training
    - safety instruction
- Community integration and involvement
    - transportation services
    - participation in community meetings
    - radio reading services (special radio transmissions for people who are blind or visually impaired that may broadcast such important material as newspaper articles and consumer information)
- Public education and outreach efforts
    - low vision fairs and seminars
    - participation in health fairs
    - distribution of public education brochures
    - presentations or other group sessions at nursing homes, senior centers, and schools
    - conferences and in-service training sessions
    - personal appearances on TV and radio promoting the Title VII, Chapter 2 program
    - newspaper articles and press releases about the benefits of vision-related services to older consumers
    - mini–adjustment training sessions
    - peer leadership training

- vocational and other training
- diabetes management training
- Equipment loan or rental and provision of assistive devices
- Evaluation and intervention
  - rehabilitation engineering
  - low vision evaluations
  - low vision and glaucoma screenings
  - in-home low vision evaluations and demonstration of low vision devices
  - visual health preventive screenings
- Psychosocial services
  - support groups for older consumers
  - individual counseling
  - telephone visitation programs
  - personal adjustment to blindness counseling
- Advocacy skills training and volunteer programs
  - Senior Companion Programs
- Outreach services
  - Outreach to unserved and underserved populations, including those for whom language, culture, or geographic barriers make access to services difficult

Many states have emphasized outreach to older persons in rural areas and minority groups who have previously had little access to vision-related rehabilitation services because of language, cultural, or geographic barriers. When funds were first available, many states used their funds to reach out to previously unserved older populations, including Native American, Hispanic, and African-American elders, and to extend services to the hard-to-reach outlying and rural areas and in many cases to the lowest-income population.

In spite of its funding limitations and its initial inequitable distribution of funds, Title VII, Chapter 2 enables agencies and states to serve older persons who were previously unserved or underserved (see Module 6).

4.1.4 Outcomes of Chapter 2 Services

The vision rehabilitation system has not as yet focused to a great extent on systematically measuring the outcomes of vision-related rehabilitation services for older persons who are blind or visually impaired. What is known about the Chapter 2 program currently relates more to the numbers of individuals served in various categories than to the impact on individual functioning (see "Costs and Benefits of the Title VII, Chapter 2 Program"). States have been asked to report the number of older persons served in specified categories of service and the number of units of service provided each year.

Not enough is known about the outcomes of service because systematic data have not been collected about the impact of these services on the lives of older individuals—what they are able to do as a result of the training they receive and how it has enhanced their lives and enabled them to regain or sustain their independence, their valued productive activities, and their involvement in community life.

Efforts are now underway to standardize data collection to measure and evaluate the outcomes of service. The need for outcome measures is discussed further in Module 6.

Costs and Benefits of the Title VII, Chapter 2 Program

- The average total state budget for the Title VII, Chapter 2 Independent Living program in FY 1995 was $248,672, including all sources of funding. Two-thirds of the funding was federal; one-third was state, in-kind, or third-party funding.
- More than 80 percent of Chapter 2 program dollars go directly to client services.
- The Chapter 2 program is serving a vulnerable and at-risk population:
  - Nearly two of every three participants in the program (64 percent) were age 76 or older; 45 percent were age 81 or older.
  - Four out of five participants (79 percent) reported one or more disabilities in addition to vision loss. The most prevalent nonvisual disabilities were cardiovascular disease, musculoskeletal disorders, diabetes, and hearing impairment.
- The average total cost per participant was approximately $540. This can be considered a good investment in preventing the high cost of falls and injury, hospital stays, and nursing home admissions; reducing the need for ongoing supportive services; and restoring older people to lives of dignity and productivity.
- Unlike the services required by older people with other disabilities, the health care system does not typically provide vision-related rehabilitation services for older persons who are blind, nor does a reimbursement funding mechanism exist for these essential services.

Source: *B. Stephens,* Independent Living Services for Individuals Who Are Blind: Annual Report for FY 1995 *(Mississippi State: Mississippi State University, Rehabilitation Research and Training Center on Blindness and Low Vision, 1996).*

MODULE 4:
COMMUNITY-BASED SERVICES
FOR OLDER PERSONS
WHO ARE BLIND
OR VISUALLY IMPAIRED

Since its inception, the Chapter 2 independent living program has had a positive impact on its participants. Professionals observe that older people show gains in their ability to organize and maintain their households, prepare and serve meals, travel safely in their homes and neighborhoods, access all forms of communication, and manage their time and financial resources (Stephens, 1996). After receiving program services, participants

- are less likely to need a personal care attendant;
- are more likely to reintegrate into community activities, and sometimes even decide to pursue paid employment; and
- feel better about themselves, their relationships with people close to them, and the future (Stephens, 1996).

Outcome data are needed to document the impact of services at their completion as well as after a specified time period—three or four months later, for example.

The following are sample case studies of consumers who were served in the Independent Living Services for Older Individuals Who Are Blind program in a rural community.* They illustrate not only the benefits for participants, but also the cost-effectiveness of services. It should be noted that the amount of funds that can be spent on adaptive equipment varies from state to state. The amounts spent in these case examples are higher than the average of $500 to $600 per consumer.

David F.

Consumer's age: 76

Disability: The report from the ophthalmologist indicated that David F. had no functional vision.

Background information: Mr. F. was a highly educated adult who lived with his wife in a retirement community. He had been told by several doctors that he would not be able to read again, and he had not been able to read any size print for more than two years. Mr. F. had

---

*These case studies were adapted with permission from Kimberly Chaffin, "Sample Success Stories: Case Studies from Consumers Served in Rural Ohio Independent Living Services for Older Individuals Who Are Blind Program," prepared for J. Scott, L. Lidoff, and A. L. Orr (Eds.), *Advocacy Tools* (New York: American Foundation for the Blind, National Aging and Vision Network, 1997).

never been exposed to rehabilitation services and was very discouraged.

Highlights of services provided: A home evaluation using lighting and magnifiers was completed by the rehabilitation teacher. It was quickly determined that with appropriate lighting and magnification, Mr. F. could read print. A closed-circuit unit was installed on his television, enabling him to read his mail and phone bills.

Total cost of services provided through Title VII, Chapter 2 funds: $1,200. Services included installing a closed-circuit television unit, improving kitchen lighting and organization, in-home training in cooking, and in-home training for writing and reading.

Rehabilitation teacher's comments: "This is a clear example of the problems with low vision services in rural areas. The closest available low vision clinic to Mr. F. is 90 minutes away. Mr. F. had not previously been informed of vision-related rehabilitation or low vision services. By completing an evaluation in Mr. F.'s home, we were able to address his home needs and eliminate much of the added time and expense of sending him 90 miles to be evaluated. The evaluation took approximately two hours of staff time, but the benefits to this consumer are immeasurable. Without Chapter 2 funds, information, advocacy, and in-home evaluation services would not exist in this state. The services that are available are generally at prohibitive cost. Low vision aids are not covered by any insurance."

Sophia M.

Consumer's age: 92

Disability: Ms. M. suffered from glaucoma and was only able to distinguish light from dark.

Background information: Ms. M. lived in her own apartment in a retirement community. A requirement for living in one's own apartment was being able to walk to the communal dining room without any assistance from staff and without disrupting any other residents. Prior to services, the staff at the retirement community were making plans to relocate Ms. M. to an assisted living area because they did not believe that she would be able to use a cane to travel on her own.

Highlights of services provided: Ms. M. received O&M training to assist her in getting to all areas within the retirement community, including her mailbox, the dining room, and a beauty shop. Advocacy services were provided to communicate to the staff about the consumer's goals and to demonstrate that she could indeed travel independently.

Total cost of services provided through Title VII, Chapter 2 funds: $900. Services included O&M training, training in writing and keeping track of telephone numbers, and training in preparing basic foods.

Rehabilitation teacher's comments: "Ms. M. would not be living in her own apartment right now without our intervention. Arrangements had already been made to move her to an assistive living environment. There are no services other than the Chapter 2 program that could have assisted this consumer in remaining independent and receiving mobility training. Now she is an inspiration to many of her peers."

Frances Q.

Consumer's age: 80

Disability: Ms. Q. developed a rare eye condition from which she suddenly lost the majority of her vision. Prior to the sudden loss, she was very independent and active in the community.

Background information: Ms. Q. owned her own home and was very active until she suddenly lost her vision. At that time, she was placed in a nursing home because she had no way of caring for herself on her own. The agency was contacted by the intermediate care facility because Ms. Q. was requesting training to return to her home.

Highlights of services provided: Training was provided to assist Ms. Q. with preparing basic meals, managing household tasks, and getting around her home safely. Safety equipment was installed in her bathroom, and an intercom was installed at the front door so that she could determine who was at the door before opening it.

Total cost of services provided through Title VII, Chapter 2 funds: $1,186. Services included O&M training; rehabilitation teaching; and installing a small microwave, improved lighting, and an intercom.

Rehabilitation teacher's comments: "When I first met Ms. Q., she was bedfast in her room in the nursing home. There were no resources other than Chapter 2 to assist her with independent living skills training to return to her own home."

Cases such as these demonstrate how a minimal investment of federal funds for independent living skills training and adaptive devices and equipment can mean the difference between continuing an essential or valued activity and giving it up, between maintaining independence and depending on others for assistance. Without these services, more costly services for in-home assistance or an even higher level of care would in all likelihood have been necessary. These cases also document the need to educate service providers in the aging network and the nursing home industry about the availability of vision-related rehabilitation services for older people and how to obtain them.

4.2 The Vision-Related Rehabilitation Service Delivery System

4.2.1 Service Delivery Structure

Specialized vision-related rehabilitation services for older persons who are blind or visually impaired are provided by professionals with special training in blindness and visual impairment. These services are offered by public and private agencies serving individuals who are blind or visually impaired, including state rehabilitation agencies, private not-for-profit rehabilitation agencies, and specialized low vision clinics.

Each state has a state vocational rehabilitation agency that provides rehabilitation services to individuals 18 years of age and older with all types of disabilities. The Rehabilitation Act gives states the right to set up a separate agency for services to people who are blind and visually impaired.

Within each state there is either a separate state agency serving people who are blind or visually impaired or a division or department within the state vocational rehabilitation agency that provides specialized vision-related rehabilitation services. Thus, the structure of vision rehabilitation services varies from state to state.

In some states, typically those with lower population density, the state agency may be the only, or the primary, vision-related rehabilitation service provider, and it may provide services directly to individuals. In other states, the state agency contracts with private agencies to provide direct services to consumers.

MODULE 4:
COMMUNITY-BASED SERVICES
FOR OLDER PERSONS
WHO ARE BLIND
OR VISUALLY IMPAIRED

State agencies also have offices at the local or regional level, but the number of these offices also varies from state to state. (For a complete listing of agencies in each state, see *AFB Directory of Services for Blind or Visually Impaired Persons in the United States and Canada,* 1997). The process of obtaining services is described in more detail in Module 5.

Since 1996, every state has received Title VII, Chapter 2 funds to provide services specifically to people age 55 and older who are blind or have severe visual impairments. Therefore, every state has funds specifically targeted for independent living skills training for older people. These services are available at no charge; costs are covered by Chapter 2 funds. Program requirements vary slightly from state to state, as does the amount of funds available for individual consumers.

Many communities also have private not-for-profit agencies that serve people who are blind or visually impaired.

Some vision-related rehabilitation services may be offered by eye care clinics, although Medicare and other health insurance policies usually do not cover these services.

4.2.2 *Specialized Services for Older Individuals*

Specialized vision-related rehabilitation services enable older persons with visual impairments to maintain a full and productive life and to maximize their ability to live independently. Essential services may be categorized as follows:

1. Training in adaptive techniques to carry out activities of daily living
   - *home and personal management skills,* such as meal preparation, personal care techniques, managing money, and labeling medications
   - *communication skills,* including the use of readers, tape recorders, large print, and/or braille for reading and writing or as an independent living skill for note taking or labeling items; computers with screen magnification; writing guides such as signature guides; telephones; and timepieces
2. *Orientation and mobility (O&M) services,* which teach safe and independent movement and travel skills, including orienting oneself in familiar and unfamiliar environments, asking for

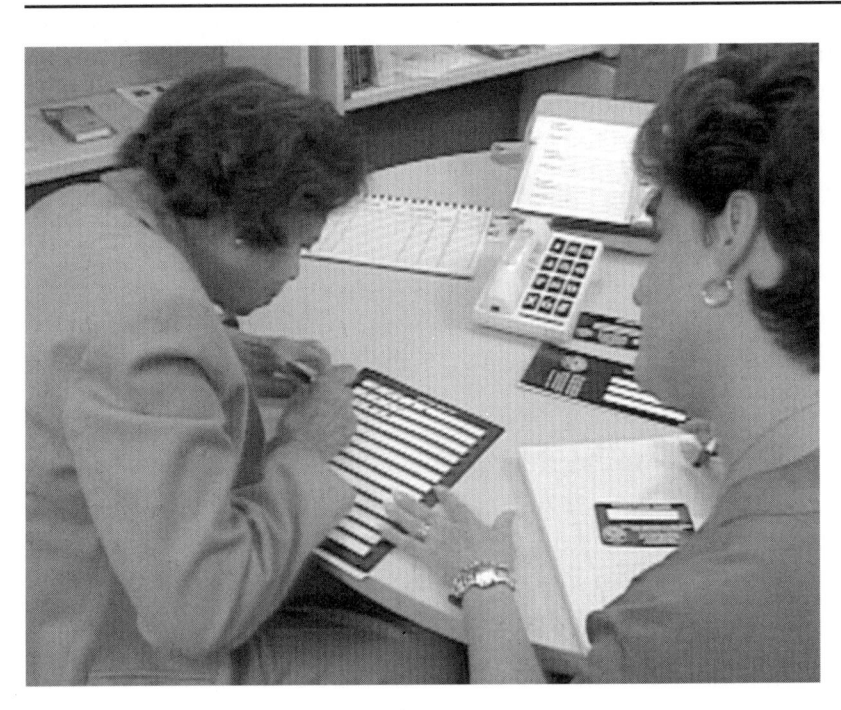

Among the specialized rehabilitation services received by older people who are visually impaired is training in adaptive techniques for everyday communication needs. This woman is learning to use various types of writing guides to write letters or notes, make out checks, and sign her name.

   assistance from others when appropriate, and moving about using a long cane or other devices
3. *Low vision services*
   - a comprehensive patient history
   - a functional low vision assessment
   - prescription of low vision devices, such as handheld magnifiers, high-intensity lamps, and other optical and nonoptical aids, designed to help the individual make the best use of remaining vision
   - instruction in the use of optical and nonoptical adaptive devices
   - follow-up instruction to ensure effective use of devices
4. *Individual counseling* to assist in the psychological and social adjustment of vision loss
5. *Support groups* to provide the opportunity to talk with others about similar problems and ways to cope

6. Teaching of skills necessary to obtain access to information and advocacy skills to gain access to mainstream community resources and services
7. Teaching of recreational and leisure-time skills to maintain social networks and participation in valued avocational activities

These services provide older people who are blind or visually impaired with the skills they need to function as independently as possible for as long as possible.

Just as physical therapy restores functioning after a person loses the use of a limb, specialized vision-related rehabilitation can restore functioning after vision loss. Whereas diagnosis and medical or surgical treatment can improve or prevent the worsening of many vision-related conditions, rehabilitative services and devices help to restore or at least improve the individual's ability to live independently.

These services can make a big difference in the life of someone who is experiencing age-related vision loss. Vision-related rehabilitation services for older persons can save older people from having to use more costly home-based long-term services through the health care and aging service systems, freeing these funds for individuals in greater need. These services can also prevent premature nursing home placement.

4.3 Specialized Vision-Related Rehabilitation Professionals

Specialized vision-related rehabilitation services are provided by a group of professionals that includes

- rehabilitation teachers;
- O&M specialists;
- low vision specialists and instructors; and
- vision rehabilitation therapists.

The sections that follow describe the work of these professionals in providing services to older people experiencing age-related vision loss; however, the role of vision rehabilitation therapists, which is a newly created specialty, is discussed under new trends in the field in Module 6.

Master's degree training is usually required for practitioners in the professions of rehabilitation teaching and O&M. (For details about rehabilitation teaching and university rehabilitation teaching programs, see Crews & Luxton, 1992; Ponchillia & Ponchillia, 1997; Wiener & Luxton, 1994; for information about O&M, see Wiener & Joffee, 1993).

4.3.1 Andragogy: Principles of Adult Learning

All vision rehabilitation professionals apply the principles of andragogy, or adult learning, in their work with adults, and particularly in work with older people who are blind or visually impaired.

The core principles of andragogy are as follows:

- The older student is the center of the teaching/learning process; the older student is always in the driver's seat.
- Teaching is goal oriented and uses a problem-solving approach.
- The teaching/learning process is mutual and reciprocal; the individual shows the instructor how she or he learns best, according to his or her years of experience.
- A step-by-step incremental presentation of skills is essential.
- Teaching must be geared to the older person's learning pace.

The rehabilitation professional needs to keep in mind that problem solving may take more time for the newly visually impaired older person, that psychological changes may affect efficiency in learning, and that "small gains" in skill acquisition and independent functioning have tremendous potential to significantly improve quality of life for the older person.

A small gain in functioning in the activities of daily living can make the difference between an older person being able to continue living in the familiar environment of his or her own home or needing to move in with a family member, consider an assistive living option, or move into a nursing home (Crews, 1991; Williams, 1984).

Two essential elements in vision rehabilitation with adults, particularly older adults, are an individualized approach and the application of andragogical principles.

4.3.2 Rehabilitation Teaching

Rehabilitation teaching is the professional discipline that teaches newly visually impaired persons the compensatory and adaptive skills that enable them to live and function independently. The goal of rehabilitation teaching is to enable these individuals to return to the level of activity enjoyed before the loss of vision. The adaptive skills needed for independent living vary considerably from person to person, requiring the teacher to possess a well-rounded and thorough knowledge of adaptive techniques for carrying out the full range of everyday tasks, as well as knowledge of adaptive devices.

The teacher also assists the individual during the adjustment process, working toward a more positive attitude about vision loss and building the motivation to take on the challenge of learning new skills and techniques. The rehabilitation teacher helps the consumer gain access to other community resources and supportive services as well.

Rehabilitation teachers generally teach the following categories of activities (Ponchillia & Ponchillia, 1997; Wiener & Luxton, 1994):

- personal management: personal hygiene, grooming, medical management, and clothing care
- communication: instruction in adaptive skills and alternative forms of reading, writing, mathematical calculation, and listening skills, as well as assistive technology
- orientation and safe movement in familiar indoor environments
- home management: general home care, kitchen skills, home repairs, and bookkeeping and financial management skills
- low vision skills: the use of remaining vision and of low vision devices and techniques
- leisure-time activities: adapted games and adaptive methods for handicrafts and active forms of recreation

The particular skills areas taught and the order in which the skills are taught are based on the older individual's life needs and interests and his or her physical ability to carry out the tasks. The older person and the rehabilitation teacher jointly develop an individualized plan for the teaching and learning of these independent living skills.

Most of the skill areas taught by rchabilitation teachers are essential for the older person to continue living and functioning independently. Although recreation and leisure activities are an area that is not necessary for survival, they significantly enhance the quality of any individual's life.

Professionals and paraprofessionals who are not trained in vision rehabilitation—such as recreation therapists, occupational therapists and occupational therapy assistants, and program staff—are frequently challenged to figure out how to include an older person who is blind or visually impaired in recreational activities with sighted peers at senior centers, adult day centers, retirement communities, or nursing homes. As the accompanying "Tips for Adapting Leisure and Recreational Activities for Individuals Who Are Blind or Visually Impaired" shows, there are several key elements to consider in planning leisure activities for older people who are visually impaired. Vision rehabilitation professionals at local agencies serving older people who are blind or visually impaired can provide consultation or in-service training for staff in community and residential settings (see Module 6).

4.3.3 Assessment, Planning, and Evaluation

The individual assessment of an older person experiencing vision loss is critical for the vision rehabilitation professional to understand from the consumer's perspective the types of skills needed to maintain or regain the best level of independent functioning. Various professionals may conduct the initial vision-related assessment of an older individual, depending on the agency structure and staffing. In many instances, the rehabilitation teacher carries out the assessment in the older person's home, which provides the opportunity to learn more about the consumer's everyday environment.

The rehabilitation professional (or other intake worker; for example, a social worker) takes a history of the consumer's background, living situation, levels of support from friends and family, and interests and hobbies and assesses how the individual handles everyday needs and activities.

Through a verbal interview, along with observation of the older person performing various activities, the rehabilitation professional assesses his or her level of functioning. From the verbal responses and activities, the professional determines the individual's eligibility for service.

Together, the older person and vision rehabilitation professional develop an individual written rehabilitation plan for the consumer's personal adjustment. They also develop an individualized plan of service related to the essential rehabilitation services needed by the

Tips for Adapting Leisure and Recreational Activities for Individuals Who Are Blind or Visually Impaired

Recreation and leisure pursuit is an important part of rehabilitation for older people with age-related vision loss. Older people with impaired vision frequently do not know that with a few modifications, they can continue their favorite leisure activities, and they also can learn new ones. Key elements of leisure and recreational activities to consider for older people include these:

- the accessibility of the activity to the individual
- the need to follow principles of adult learning in teaching the activity.
- the visual requirements of a particular individual
- whether the individual has other sensory losses or physical disabilities that affect participation
- the participant's interest in a particular activity and motivation for participating

Some strategies for adapting activities for older people who are blind or visually impaired include the following:

- Substitute touch techniques to replace observation of the instructor when teaching an activity.
- Verbalize instructions and provide narration during the activity.
- Introduce adaptive equipment such as a low vision device, braille or taped materials, or adapted games. Bingo, checkers, and playing cards are available in braille and large print.
- Acquaint the individual with audiodescribed videotapes and television programs, where available, in which the visual portion of a performance is described by a special narrator. The describer gives the overall visual picture, explains subtle facial gestures and nuances, and describes the setting for the benefit of the person who has low vision or is blind.
- Work to break down or eliminate barriers and negative attitudes about the individual's ability to participate in leisure activities, such as the following:

  - lack of personal mobility
  - lack of transportation
  - lack of knowledge of the activities
  - lack of motivation
  - fear of seeming inadequate or incapable

In-service training for recreation therapists, community recreational staff, and program staff at senior centers can help them to integrate the individual who is blind or visually impaired into ongoing activities and programming.

individual. The consumer is at the center of the service plan and the delivery of services.

Thus, for example, if an older individual was accustomed to preparing meals, handling correspondence, and carrying out other household chores prior to vision loss, the teacher would encourage and provide instruction in adaptive techniques in each of these activities.

Some older individuals may opt to learn braille as an alternative to maintaining print records (see "Braille Instruction and Braille Literacy"). Others may use large print, and still others may choose to use cassette tape.

Some individuals may have simplified their meals preparation even before any loss of vision to consist primarily of frozen foods and canned goods. These older people may want only to learn labeling techniques so they can identify the contents of their various cans and packages. Individuals who have enjoyed cooking may want more extensive training in the use of kitchen appliances and techniques for measuring, pouring, and cutting.

The teacher also needs to help the older individual who is blind or visually impaired to solve problems related to vision loss and identify community resources. If the older person typically drove to church, how else can he or she get there? If she or he enjoyed shopping or needs to shop for groceries, what resources are available to help this older individual continue to accomplish this task independently?

Braille Instruction and Braille Literacy

Braille literacy has been a prominent issue in the field of blindness and visual impairment in the 1990s as it relates to the education of children who are blind or severely visually impaired and for adults who want to learn braille as a means of reading and writing or as an independent living skill. Teaching braille and its uses to older persons experiencing age-related vision loss also deserves consideration.

Many older people can benefit from learning grade 1 braille (the alphabet) so that they can jot down a telephone number or label an item in braille, for example, rather than using braille as a primary form of literacy—to read an entire book or as a primary means of written communication. In this sense, braille is an independent living skill.

Because the task of teaching is time consuming, it is often difficult for agencies to allocate staff time for teaching braille. In addition, older people who have neuropathy may not be able to read braille because of the lack of sensitivity in their fingertips.

If an older person wants to learn braille and is capable of doing so, however, then it is important to provide access to instruction. Older people should not be told that they do not need to learn braille or that they are too old to learn. If agency-based instruction is not possible, a correspondence course is available through various sources, such as the Hadley School in Illinois (see the Resources at the end of this module), for individuals who can work independently.

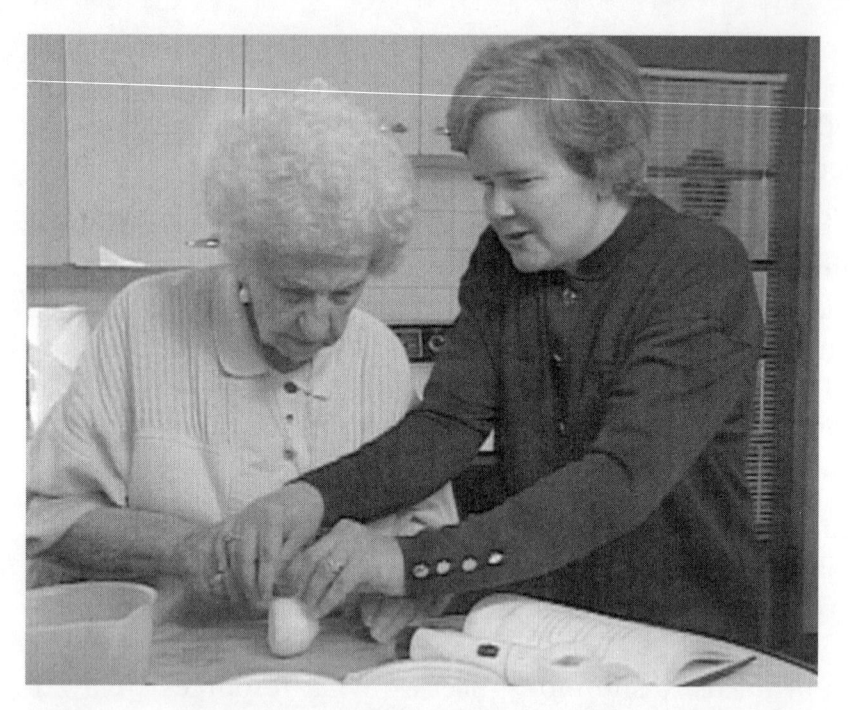

MODULE 4:
COMMUNITY-BASED SERVICES
FOR OLDER PERSONS
WHO ARE BLIND
OR VISUALLY IMPAIRED

Rehabilitation teachers can train older people who are blind or visually impaired in adaptive cooking techniques, such as safe ways to cut and dice an onion.

The magnitude of an individual's accomplishment in rehabilitation is best judged from the individual's perspective. An important principle in all situations is that by mastering a technique, the individual regains a sense of mastery over his or her own personal situation. This gain in self-confidence helps to break any cycle of dependency that may have begun when the older person experienced a loss of vision and began to rely on family, community support services, or institutional care for activities previously performed independently.

4.3.4 Orientation and Mobility

O&M is the professional discipline that involves teaching people who are blind or visually impaired how to become oriented to the indoor and outdoor environment and to travel outdoors. These skills include the use of a long cane, sophisticated electronic travel aids, and the use of public transit. The O&M specialist also provides counseling to increase confidence and motivation.

The overreaching goal of O&M instruction is to enable the older individual to return to the level of mobility that he or she experienced before the onset of blindness or visual impairment. Individual characteristics, attributes, and physical abilities, rather than age, are usually the factors in determining mobility goals that individuals set for themselves.

For example, if an individual was accustomed to walking to church before experiencing any vision problems, this activity will likely become a goal that the instructor and the individual will work on achieving, and the instruction will be tailored accordingly. That is, special attention will be given to the route from the older person's home to church.

If, on the other hand, the individual was accustomed to walking only as far as the community room in his or her retirement center, then this destination will probably become a mobility goal for this individual, and training would again be tailored accordingly. For example, special attention would be given to learning to operate an elevator.

Thus, O&M specialists provide varying levels of instruction, depending on the individual with whom they are working. As with rehabilitation teaching, the magnitude of the consumer's accomplishment can best be judged from the individual's perspective.

4.3.5 Low Vision Services

The low vision specialist is an ophthalmologist or optometrist with a specialization in low vision. This professional provides comprehensive low vision services, including the following:

- a comprehensive patient history
- a functional low vision assessment
- prescription of low vision devices
- instruction in the use of low vision devices
- follow-up services

Vision rehabilitation professionals can also provide instruction in the use of some prescribed low vision devices, such as magnifiers, CCTVs, or telescopes. For more details about the low vision examination and services, see Module 2.

Many older people still do not know about low vision services, particularly individuals living outside major metropolitan areas. Although low vision services are becoming more widely available throughout the country, in some states the availability of certified providers for comprehensive low vision services is extremely limited. Low-income older people, members of minority groups, and those living in rural areas in particular have limited access to low vision services and eye care in general.

In addition to the need for greater availability of low vision services, more attention to the follow-up component of low vision rehabilitation remains critical if older consumers are to make maximum use of their prescribed low vision devices, such as handheld magnifiers, telescopes, and high-intensity lighting. Rehabilitation teachers and other vision rehabilitation professionals are also trained to carry out the follow-up phase of low vision services, to enhance the ability of programs to provide sufficient follow-through in the effective use of these devices. Vision rehabilitation agencies need to give increasing priority to the follow-up phase of instruction in the use of devices, even when the agency does not provide the low vision evaluation, so that fewer devices go unused because individuals become frustrated and conclude that "they just don't work" (see Module 2).

Agencies serving people who are visually impaired and that offer low vision services, as well as low vision clinics under other auspices, need to work to bring these services into community settings.

For example, one low vision clinic developed a community-based low vision service delivery model to reach frail African-American elders. In cooperation with a community development organization owned and managed by African-Americans, the low vision clinic brought low vision screening into community centers in African-American communities to evaluate this largely unserved group. The community development organization raised funds to support the costs of the low vision services for every older person who needed them. Through this method, individuals with undiagnosed glaucoma and diabetic retinopathy that might otherwise have gone undetected and untreated were identified and served.

4.4 Rehabilitation Teaching Methods and Learning Environments

The field of vision rehabilitation has worked for the last three decades to find the most effective methods of rehabilitation and the most conducive environments for learning for older people. The continuum of methods ranges from a stay of several weeks at a rehabilitation center for training, to training in a community agency, to carrying out assessment and instruction in the older person's home. Each has merits; agency-based training, whether in a rehabilitation center or in the individual's community, and home-based training both offer advantages for different groups of older individuals.

Deciding which learning environment to emphasize or whether to offer both can be determined only through a comprehensive assessment of the population of older people who are visually impaired in the agency's service area, by the geographic factors involved, and by an audit of the agency's resources, particularly personnel and funding. An exemplary model would provide both agency-based and home-based rehabilitation teaching and O&M services.

4.4.1 Home-Based Model

The majority of vision rehabilitation agencies currently use a home-based model. This model is particularly important to reach older consumers who would otherwise not go to an agency for services because of geographic distances from the agency, transportation difficulties, limiting physical conditions, or chronic health problems.

The home-based model has other advantages. It allows older consumers to learn adaptive skills in the primary environment in which they will be used, and it allows the service provider to tailor instruction to the individual's style and pace of learning in a familiar environment. Gerontologists have found that older people learn best in a familiar and comfortable environment.

This method also enables rehabilitation professionals to assess the older person's environment and to make suggestions for environmental modifications that would enhance the individual's independent functioning and ensure safety.

If family members are at home while their older relative is learning new skills, they can participate in the training or learn about the new skills through observation.

The major disadvantage of the home-based model of rehabilitation is that it does not give the older individual the opportunity to meet peers who are experiencing some of the same challenges and frustrations associated with adjustment to vision loss.

4.4.2 Agency-Based Model

The agency-based model of rehabilitation services provides another, equally important, array of advantages. In general, more time can be spent on learning skills. Clients can typically come to an agency more frequently than the rehabilitation teacher can get to each individual's home, especially in non-urban communities.

In an agency serving blind and visually impaired persons, skills may be taught in a group environment that provides for mutual learning and sharing, and many agencies provide support groups in which consumers can share their experiences, frustrations, and successes in learning new skills. Participation in group rehabilitation services offers the older person the opportunity to learn with others, to perceive that others may also have difficulties mastering new skills, and to learn from their peers as well as from the instructor. The social environment and opportunities to establish a new social network are extremely valuable during the adjustment process.

The major disadvantage of agency-based training is that the learner must transfer new knowledge and skills from the learning environment to the environment in which the skills will be used on a routine basis. For some older people who may have difficulty learning and using adaptive skills, transferring to a different environment can affect the ability to use the skill.

4.4.3 Combined Model

The ideal model is to offer older consumers choices about the skills they need and the best learning environment for them as individuals. Providing services in more than one environment by more than one method also ensures that services are accessible and amenable to a larger group of consumers.

A combined model of service delivery offers initial instruction in an agency setting through individual and/or group instruction, followed by in-home instruction as needed. The combined model benefits older consumers who have the opportunity to experience both types of teaching approaches and learning environments.

The demand for services and the cost of service delivery both affect the way that agencies develop their service delivery methods. For example, many agencies convert to agency-based group teaching methods to reduce their growing waiting lists of older consumers or to make maximum use of limited Chapter 2 funds and limited personnel. The secondary gains to consumers of meeting and learning with others encourage some agencies to continue to offer the agency-based group teaching method in addition to in-home services after group instruction.

The efficiency and cost-effectiveness of home-based or agency-based vision rehabilitation services must be weighed against the realities of ensuring that older persons have access to resources and services. One key factor is the availability of transportation services, which make it possible for many consumers to attend the community-based agency for independent living skills training. Although some agencies have their own vehicles or access to community vehicles, lack of door-to-door or accessible transportation is a major barrier to services in many areas.

Follow-up services provided in the consumer's home by the rehabilitation teacher are an essential component of learning skills in an agency setting to ensure that the older person is able to transfer skills learned in the agency setting to the home environment.

As a result of the continuing growth in the population of older people who are blind or visually impaired, vision rehabilitation is a growing and changing field. Module 5 discusses ways of improving the access of older individuals to these services, and Module 6 examines current issues and trends in delivering vision-related rehabilitation services against the background of this ongoing change.

References

AFB directory of services for blind or visually impaired persons in the United States and Canada (25th ed.). (1997). New York: AFB Press.

Crews, J. (1991, September 23). *The needs of older people who are blind in the United States: A background report for the reauthorization of Title VII Part C of the Rehabilitation Act.* Saginaw: Michigan Commission for the Blind.

Crews, J. E., & Luxton, L. (1992). Rehabilitation teaching for older adults. In A. L. Orr, *Vision and aging: Crossroads for service delivery.* (pp. 233–253). New York: American Foundation for the Blind.

Herndon, G. (1993). *Analysis of Title VII, Part C, independent living services for older Americans with visual impairments, fiscal year 1991–92.* Mississippi State: Mississippi State University, Rehabilitation Research and Training Center on Blindness and Low Vision.

Moore, E. J., & Stephens, B. (1995). *Analysis of Title VII, Part C, independent living services for older Americans with visual impairments, fiscal year 1994.* Mississippi State: Mississippi State University Rehabilitation Research & Training Center on Blindness and Low Vision.

Ponchillia, P. E., & Ponchillia, S. V. (1997). *Foundations of rehabilitation teaching with persons who are blind or visually impaired.* New York: AFB Press.

Stephens, B. (1994). *Analysis of Title VII, Chapter 2, independent living services for older Americans with visual impairments, fiscal year 1992–1993.* Mississippi State: Mississippi State University, Rehabilitation Research and Training Center on Blindness and Low Vision.

Stephens, B. (1996). *Independent living services for older individuals who are blind: Annual report for FY 1995.* Mississippi State: Mississippi State University, Rehabilitation Research and Training Center on Blindness and Low Vision.

Wiener, W. R., & Joffee, E. (1993). The O&M personnel shortage and university training programs. *RE:view, 25*(2), 67–73.

Wiener, W. R., & Luxton, L. (1994). The development of guidelines for university programs in rehabilitation teaching. *RE:view, 26*(1), 7–14.

Williams, T. F. (Ed.). (1984). *Rehabilitation in the aging.* New York: Raven.

RECOMMENDED TEACHING METHODS

Lecture

Provide an overview of the core services of vision rehabilitation (the Title VII Chapter 2 federally funded program for older persons who are blind) and the professionals who provide the services.

Guest Speakers

Invite guest speakers from public and private agencies serving older blind and visually impaired persons to describe how the public (state) rehabilitation agency and its local offices determine eligibility for initiating services and to describe the services of the private agency.

Small-Group Brainstorming

Organize students into small groups and ask them to develop a plan to integrate older people who are visually impaired into a community senior center.

Have the groups brainstorm about the elements of a needs assessment and an assessment of what older visually impaired persons want after their rehabilitation.

Field Trip: Agency Visit

As time and resources permit, accompany students to visit a vision rehabilitation agency so that they may fully understand the nature of service delivery. This visit can be scheduled in addition to or instead of having guest lectures in the classroom. One recommended approach is to have a guest from the state or public agency, and have students visit a private agency.

RESOURCES

Recommended Readings

Crews, J. E., & Luxton, L. (1992). Rehabilitation teaching for older adults. In A. L. Orr, *Vision and aging: Crossroads for service delivery.* (pp. 233–253). New York: American Foundation for the Blind.

Dickman, I. (1983). *Making life more livable.* New York: American Foundation for the Blind.

Griffin-Shirley, N., & Groff, G. (1994). *Prescriptions for independence: Working with older people who are visually impaired.* New York: AFB Press.

Orr, A. L. (1992). An overview of the blindness system. In A. L. Orr (Ed.), *Vision and aging: Crossroads for service delivery* (pp. 159–183). New York: American Foundation for the Blind.

Paskin, N., & Soucy-Moloney, L. A. (1995). *Whatever works: Confident living for people with impaired vision.* New York: The Lighthouse.

Ringgold, M. (1991). *Out of the corner of my eye.* New York: American Foundation for the Blind.

MODULE 4:
COMMUNITY-BASED SERVICES
FOR OLDER PERSONS
WHO ARE BLIND
OR VISUALLY IMPAIRED

Further Reading

Crews, J. (1991, September 23). *The needs of older people who are blind in the United States: A background report for the reauthorization of Title VII Part C of the Rehabilitation Act.* Saginaw: Michigan Commission for the Blind.

Crews, J. E., & Clark, H. C. (1997). Orientation and mobility for the older person. In B. B. Blasch, W. R. Wiener, & R. L. Welsh (Eds.), *Foundations of orientation and mobility* (2nd ed.) (pp. 439–455). New York: AFB Press.

Crudden, A. (1995). Service delivery to older people who are blind. *RE:view, 27,*(3), 123–129.

Moore, J., & Stephens, B. (1994). Independent living services for older individuals who are blind: Issues and practices. *American Rehabilitation, 20*(1), 30–34.

Nelson, K. A., & Dimitrova, E. (1993). Statistical brief #36, severe visual impairment in the United States and in each state, *Journal of Visual Impairment & Blindness, 87*(3), 80–85.

Stephens, B. (1995). *Analysis of Title VII, Chapter 2—Independent living services for older individuals who are blind—fiscal year 1994.* Mississippi State: Mississippi State University, Rehabilitation Research and Training Center on Blindness and Low Vision.

Yeadon, A. (1984). The informal care group: Problem or potential? *Journal of Visual Impairment & Blindness, 78,* 149–154.

Other Materials

Aging and Vision (1996). New York: The Lighthouse.

This five-volume series is designed for consumers and their families and professionals serving older people who are blind or visually impaired. Jointly distributed by The Lighthouse and the American Foundation for the Blind, it may be purchased separately or as a set. The five components of the series are as follows:

> *Critical Concerns and Effective Practices: Final Focus Group Report* presents the findings of five national focus groups that met in 1993 and 1994 to define critical concerns about vision rehabilitation programs for older people who experience severe visual impairment. The 87 participants included directors of programs funded under Title VII, Chapter 2 of the Rehabilitation Act; directors and senior staff of private agencies serving older persons with impaired vision; repre-

sentatives of the aging network, medicine, academia, optometry, ophthalmology, and various social service agencies; and consumers. A common finding was that the intensity and comprehensiveness of vision rehabilitation services for older people frequently reflect the resources available to each organization, rather than the need for services. The report also details some effective practice strategies used by organizations serving older people with impaired vision.

The Directory of Programs and Services for Older People with Impaired Vision lists services by state, provides a general description of services, includes regional and national programs, and includes a glossary of commonly used vision terms. The large-print format and the design promote accessibility to people with impaired vision.

The VisualEyes Curriculum on vision rehabilitation is targeted to health and human service workers who are not eye care specialists. It offers an approach to understanding the basics of vision rehabilitation, with specific attention to the needs of older adults. Details are also provided on how to structure the training, recruit the audience, and locate faculty.

The VisualEyes Workbook is designed to help people use the information they received from the VisualEyes training in the workplace. A topical outline of the curriculum and glossary of terminology are provided, and worksheets used in all training activities are also included.

Creative Solutions to Program Needs reviews programs in the aging and vision rehabilitation networks from across the country serving older people who are blind or visually impaired. The emphasis is on the historical development, funding, effective strategies, consumer involvement, and the use of volunteers.

The Functional Vision Screening Questionnaire. (1996). New York: The Lighthouse.

The questionnaire is a screening tool that identifies older people who may be experiencing a vision problem and who would benefit from seeing an optometrist or ophthalmologist. The 15-item questionnaire is available in English, Spanish, Italian, German, French, Polish, and Chinese. It may be filled out independently by an older adult or administered by an interviewer. Details on scoring and interpreting the results are included. Each questionnaire is produced in pads of 25.

The Lighthouse National Survey on Vision Loss: The experience, attitudes and knowledge of middle-aged and older Americans. (1995.) New York: The Lighthouse.

Organizations

The organizations listed here are just a few of the many that offer services and referrals to help older individuals who are blind or visually impaired live independent lives in their communities. For referrals to vision rehabilitation services, consult the vision-related organizations listed in the Resources section at the end of Module 2 and the *AFB Directory of Services for Blind and Visually Impaired Persons in the United States and Canada,* published by AFB Press.

Administration on Aging
U.S. Department of Health and Human Services
200 Independence Avenue, S.W.
Washington, DC 20201
(202) 401-4634, or (800) 677-1116 (Eldercare Locator)
www.aoa.dhhs.gov

Acts as an advocate within the federal government for elderly persons. Administers the Older Americans Act of 1965 to assist states and local communities in developing comprehensive service systems for older persons. Operates the Eldercare Locator, a national toll-free information and assistance directory, at (800) 677-1116, for older people and caregivers, which provides the name and telephone number of the nearest Area Agency on Aging.

Hadley School for the Blind
700 Elm Street
Winnetka, IL 60093-0299, USA
(847) 446-8111 or (800) 323-4238
FAX: (847) 446-9916

Provides tuition-free home studies, including a correspondence course for learning braille.

Lighthouse National Center for Vision and Aging
11 East 59th Street
New York, NY 10022

(212) 821-9200 or (800) 334-5497 or TDD (212) 821-9713
FAX: (212) 821-9705
http://www.lighthouse.org

Serves as a national clearinghouse for information on vision and aging and referrals for services.

National Association of Area Agencies on Aging
1112 16th Street, N.W., Suite 100
Washington, DC 20036
(202) 296-8130
FAX: (202) 296-8134
E-mail: jjfn4a@erols.com

Provides referrals to local Area Agencies on Aging.

National Association of Radio Reading Services
2100 Wharton Street, Suite 140
Pittsburgh, PA 15203
(412) 488-3944
FAX: (412) 488-3953

Provides information on and promotes radio reading services. Has closed-circuit radio broadcasts of daily newspapers plus other materials. Maintains a circulating library of books and programs on tape. Publishes *Hearsay Newsletter* and *Directory of Radio Reading Services.*

National Library Service for the Blind and Visually Handicapped
Library of Congress
1291 Taylor Street, N.W.
Washington, DC 20542
(800) 424-8567

Provides free library services to people with vision problems. Offers braille and large-print materials, recorded books, and other periodicals.

Resources for Rehabilitation
33 Bedford Street, Suite 19A
Lexington, MA 02173
(617) 862-6455
FAX: (617) 861-7517

Provides training and information to professionals and the public about the needs of individuals with disabilities and the resources

MODULE 4:
COMMUNITY-BASED SERVICES
FOR OLDER PERSONS
WHO ARE BLIND
OR VISUALLY IMPAIRED

available to meet those needs. Publications include the Living with Low Vision Series and large-print publications.

Vision Foundation
818 Mt. Auburn Street
Watertown, MA 02172
(617) 926-4232
FAX: (617) 926-1412

Provides information and publications in adapted formats for adults coping with vision loss. Publishes the Vision Resource List, which includes information on special products and services for people with visual impairments.

FACT SHEET

Independent Living Services for Older Individuals Who Are Blind Program

(Title VII, Chapter 2 of the Rehabilitation Act)

The 1978 amendments of the Rehabilitation Act of 1973 added a new section that authorized grants to state vocational rehabilitation agencies to provide independent living services to older blind and visually impaired persons.

For purposes of this program, the term *older individual who is blind* is defined as "an individual age 55 or older whose severe visual impairment makes competitive employment extremely difficult to attain but for whom independent living goals are feasible."

A wide variety of services may be provided through this program, including training in skills of daily living, provision of adaptive aids and appliances, low vision services, orientation and mobility (O&M) training, training in communication skills, family and peer counseling, and community integration (including outreach and information and referral).

Each state designs its own program to meet the specific needs of its population of older people who are blind or visually impaired. Many states have emphasized outreach to rural older persons and minority groups who have previously had little access to vision-related rehabilitation services.

The Chapter 2 program has a positive impact on participants. Data indicates that participants' independent living skills improve substantially. They show gains in their ability to organize and maintain their households, prepare and serve meals, travel safely in their homes and neighborhoods, access all forms of communication, and manage their time and financial resources.

After receiving program services, participants are less likely to need a personal care attendant and are more likely to resume community activities and sometimes even decide to pursue paid employment. They feel better about themselves, their relationships with people close to them, and the future.

More than 80 percent of Chapter 2 program dollars go directly to client services.

The average total cost reported per program participant is $500 to $600.

Title VII, Chapter 2 has enabled agencies and states to serve older persons who were previously unserved or underserved. In particular, it allows agencies to reach out to previously unserved older populations such as African-American, American Indian, and Hispanic elders and to extend services to the hard-to-reach outlying and rural areas, and in many cases, to the lowest-income population.

Adapted from material prepared by Lorraine Lidoff, National Program Associate on Aging, American Foundation for the Blind, and Barry C. Stephens, Research Scientist, Programs for Older Blind, Mississippi State University Rehabilitation Research and Training Center on Blindness and Low Vision, November 1996.

Copyright © 1998, AFB Press

MODULE 5

Improving Access to Vision Rehabilitation and Support Services

Access to services is a critical issue for older people who experience age-related vision loss. Services can only be as good as the access an individual has to them. Great strides have been made in the last decade, both in the availability of vision-related services to older people and in the education of service providers and the general public about their existence. Despite this progress, many older people and their family members are still unaware that these vital services exist, that they are eligible for them, and that there are effective ways of gaining access to them.

It should be noted, however, that it is also important for primary care physicians, eye care professionals, and service providers in the aging network and allied health fields to be familiar with the vision-related rehabilitation field in order to improve access to both vision rehabilitation and supportive services from the aging network. That is, to continue to live independently in their own homes, older people who are visually impaired may need other kinds of assistance and support in addition to specialized vision-related rehabilitation services, such as Meals on Wheels, door-to-door transportation to medical appointments, or a reader to manage bills and other mail. It is equally important, therefore, that service providers understand that home- and community-based long-term services are essential resources for older people, so that access to these services can also be enhanced.

Topic Outline

5.1 Barriers to Effective Service Delivery
- **5.1.1** Barriers in the Service Delivery System
- **5.1.2** Language, Cultural, and Economic Barriers
- **5.1.3** Environmental and Geographic Barriers
- **5.1.4** Funding Limitations
- **5.1.5** Attitudinal Barriers
- **5.1.6** Limited Information about Services
- **5.1.7** Efforts to Remove Barriers to Services

5.2 Access to Vision Rehabilitation Services
- **5.2.1** Eligibility for Vision-Related Rehabilitation Services
- **5.2.2** Obtaining Services
- **5.2.3** Effective Referrals
- **5.2.4** Follow-Up and Follow-Through

5.3 Home- and Community-Based Long-Term Services
- **5.3.1** The Aging Network and HCBC
- **5.3.2** Vision Rehabilitation and HCBC
- **5.3.3** Improving Access to HCBC Services

5.4 Access to Services in Nursing Homes

5.5 An Eye Toward the Future

Learner Objectives

1. The student will be able to identify the individual and societal barriers that make it difficult for older adults with age-related vision loss to obtain the vision-related services they need in order to continue to live as independently as possible.

2. The student will be able to describe how he or she, as a professional, can break down some of the systemic and attitudinal barriers to the delivery of vision-related services.

3. The student will be able to describe the eligibility criteria for vision rehabilitation services for older adults, how to gain access to the services, and the range of available services.

MODULE 5:
IMPROVING ACCESS
TO VISION REHABILITATION
AND SUPPORT SERVICES

4. The student will be able to describe how to make effective referrals for vision-related services.

5. The student will be able to describe ways to ensure that older clients who are visually impaired have access to home- and community-based long-term services through the aging network and health care system.

5.1 Barriers to Effective Service Delivery

No matter how effective a service is, it can only be successful if the people who need it are aware of its existence and are able to make use of it.

The demographics of aging and vision have begun to shape public policy in the area of aging and age-related vision loss that has, in turn, affected the availability of services. Funding increased steadily during the late 1990s for the Title VII, Chapter 2 Independent Living Services for Older Individuals Who Are Blind program (see Module 4), although not nearly enough. Vision-related rehabilitation services are now available in every state, although they are not yet equitably distributed in concert with the distribution of older visually impaired persons around the country.

Even though considerable progress has been made in the last decade in improving access to vision-related services, a number of factors still prevent many people who are eligible for these services from obtaining them. In order to improve access to services for older people who are blind or visually impaired, it is important to understand and eliminate the particular barriers to service.

In general, however, it is important that legislation keep pace with the exponential growth in this population and that agencies serving people who are blind or visually impaired make service delivery to older persons a priority.

Professionals in the aging network and the vision rehabilitation field need to get to know each other and work together to ensure that funding and services are available for their mutual client population. (This is discussed in more detail in Module 7.) They need to form effective collaborative partnerships so that older people can receive comprehensive and holistic vision-related rehabilitation and supportive services. The arenas of aging and disability must seek to build common ground, educating each other, joining forces, and, in times of scarce funding, maximizing resources that may become strained or more inadequate in the face of the growing population of older persons.

5.1.1 Barriers in the Service Delivery System

Professionals in the aging and disability arenas, including vision rehabilitation, have not always known a great deal about each other's services, funding streams, eligibility criteria, or mode of operation. This reality has impeded access to services for older clients, because individuals who are receiving services in one system may not be referred for appropriate services to the other (Biegel, Petchers, Snyder, & Beisgin, 1989; Stuen, 1991).

Efforts have been made during the 1990s, however, to increase understanding and interaction between the two systems. In many states, Title VII, Chapter 2 (Independent Living Services for Older Individuals Who Are Blind) program staff and their counterparts in the aging network have established formal and informal cooperative agreements that set out procedures and projects for cooperation between agencies. Collaborative efforts have taken place at the federal, state, and local levels to improve service delivery by breaking down these barriers. (This is discussed in detail in Module 7.)

5.1.2 Language, Cultural, and Economic Barriers

At the local level, agencies need to know the pockets of the older population that are not being served. If particular groups of potential clients are not seeking services, agencies must investigate the possibility that specific barriers are preventing them from accessing the service delivery system.

For example, it has been documented that the incidence of glaucoma is higher among African-Americans, and diabetic retinopathy is higher among African-Americans, Hispanics, and American Indians (National Advisory Eye Council, 1993; see Module 2). Geographic, language, or cultural factors may make it difficult for many older persons in these groups to seek services.

When consumers are not seeking services, agencies need to identify and imple\ment strategies that will bring services to them in the familiar environment of their immediate community, such as employing bilingual and bicultural staff and implementing outreach programs (see Module 6).

In low-income communities, access to any form of high-quality and affordable health care is often limited. Because vision loss is not life threatening, it can easily be overlooked or ignored by the aging individual and family members and even by medical professionals.

5.1.3 Environmental and Geographic Barriers

In many parts of the country, especially in rural communities, older people and their family members have significantly limited access to information about rehabilitation services and to the services themselves, simply by virtue of their geographic distance from these services.

Transportation is the critical access service for many older people, but it is limited in many different environments, including major urban areas. When services are not in their immediate community, individuals are also typically less aware that the services exist and are not knowledgeable about what they offer.

5.1.4 Funding Limitations

As has been noted in other modules, there are limited sources of funding for vision rehabilitation services for older individuals experiencing age-related vision loss. Title VII, Chapter 2 of the Rehabilitation Act of 1973—the Independent Living Services for Older Individuals Who Are Blind program—is the only federally, publicly funded program targeted specifically for the approximately 5 million older persons experiencing age-related vision loss (see Module 4). Moreover, vision-related rehabilitation services traditionally have not been reimbursable through the health care system, although attempts are being made to acquire third-party reimbursement for vision-related services and to move vision rehabilitation into the health care arena (Lidoff, 1997; Massof, 1996; see Module 6). These limitations in funding make it difficult both for agencies to pay for the provision of services and for individuals to afford the services that they need.

5.1.5 Attitudinal Barriers

Negative attitudes and stereotypes about older people, blindness, and disabilities in general remain common in our society, and frequently stand in the way of older people's obtaining the services they need. Among the attitudinal barriers to service are the following:

- Ageism, or a stereotypic view of older people as having a limited capacity to function as productive individuals, is still prevalent in society.
- Negative attitudes about the capabilities of individuals with disabilities are also common. Lack of exposure to high-functioning, capable individuals who have disabilities, especially blindness, helps to perpetuate such stereotypic thinking. It is extremely important to dispel the myths that abound in this society about people who have disabilities.
- Another outdated assumption is that blind people who work can perform only certain types of jobs, such as running newspaper stands or similar concessions, or working in facility-based employment (what used to be called sheltered workshops) making mops and brooms. Many older people themselves grew up with stereotypic images of people who were blind as beggars with a tin cup selling pencils. Today, through assistive technology, job modification, and rehabilitation services, many visually impaired people can continue to perform the same jobs they had before they experienced vision loss.
- Some service providers still have stereotypic attitudes about older people who are blind or visually impaired, the abilities of such individuals to function independently, their need for assistance, or their ability to participate alongside their sighted peers.

Many people, including service professionals, all too often focus on what the older blind or visually impaired person will not be able to do, how it is dangerous for older people with impaired vision to perform the same activities as their sighted peers, and how difficult it is to serve them.

Such stereotypic thinking can result in the "whose-client-is-this-anyway?" syndrome; and the answer has often been, "Somebody else's." For example, if an individual who is seeking home care is blind, a service provider at a home care agency or an agency serving elderly persons may automatically refer the client to an agency in the vision field, without thinking about the nature of the service that is required and whether it is related to blindness or to illness or general frailty. For example, professionals in the aging network as well as consumers and their family members frequently contact an agency serving people who are blind or visually impaired to request home care or assistance for a visually impaired older person. They assume that since the individual is blind or severely visually impaired, the vision field must provide the full range of services needed, whether the services are vision related or not. Although many older people who are visually impaired may in fact need home care based on the complexity of their health and physical condition, that service is not provided by the vision rehabilitation system.

To understand under whose auspices a service is provided, it helps to know the funding sources and the legislation and regulations governing it. Increasing the awareness of service providers about the kinds of assistance that agencies serving individuals who are visually impaired can provide can help them determine which service delivery system is responsible for delivering a particular service.

Older people often have their own attitudinal barriers that can interfere with obtaining services, such as the following:

- difficulty admitting to themselves and others that they have a problem because it may be the first sign of aging
- reluctance to seek assistance from an agency that has the word "blind" in its name, either because they are afraid to admit to having a visual impairment or because they do not think the impairment is severe enough to warrant that description (Many people assume that the services are strictly for people who are totally blind if an agency has the word "blind" in its name. For this reason, among others, the words "and visually impaired" have been added to the names of many agencies "for the blind.")
- feelings of self-consciousness or embarrassment about using assistive devices in public
- stereotypic perceptions about disability in general and blindness in particular, based on outdated images from their youth
- cultural images of the individual with a disability as someone to be either revered or shunned
- stereotypic thinking about the prescribed roles for older people, for individuals of all ages who are blind, and particularly for older people who are blind or visually impaired
- belief that vision loss is an inevitable part of the aging process and that there is therefore no point in seeking services, including eye care
- association of vision-related rehabilitation services with the receipt of welfare, which the older person may resist
- the conclusion that because nothing can be done medically in a particular case to restore lost vision, that living independently is

impossible. It is often difficult for an older person to hear beyond the pronouncement of his or her vision loss, even if the eye care professional or other service providers have provided additional information about other assistance that is available.

Vision loss can have a significant negative effect on the older individual's sense of self-worth and self-confidence (see Module 3). It can contribute significantly to the cycle of failing to seek services or needed care—and in turn becoming more dependent and feeling worse about oneself.

Vision-related rehabilitation services need to become an accepted part of the continuum of services, rather than being so separate and stigmatizing that older people feel resistant to seeking and accepting help from appropriate agencies.

5.1.6 Limited Information About Services

Many older people and their family members still do not know where to go for help when age-related vision loss occurs. They need access to information. They need to know that the services exist, their eligibility criteria, and how to gain access to these services.

People who come into contact with an older person who is visually impaired—including friends and family members as well as service providers in the aging network and health system—need to understand the issues associated with age-related vision loss. It is important for them to realize that vision loss can be a life crisis for someone who has lived 60, 70, or 80 years as a sighted person.

Information about the psychosocial aspects of vision loss would help friends and relatives understand and know how to respond when the older person is going through a difficult time psychologically (see Module 3 for more details.) For example, a family member's benevolent attempts to "take care of" his or her older relative can lead to unnecessary dependence (sometimes termed "learned helplessness") on the part of that older relative.

5.1.7 Efforts to Remove Barriers to Services

Because many of the barriers to obtaining vision-related services for older individuals relate to a general lack of information, misunderstanding, and misperception about age-related vision loss, public education and outreach services are crucial to improving access to these services. Thus, in addition to focusing on the provision of services, professionals in the vision rehabilitation field are aggressively tackling two essential activities, which are

- public and professional education to disperse information about aging and vision loss to a wide audience; and
- targeted outreach efforts to ensure that older people—particularly those in high-risk groups such as Hispanic, African-American, Asian, and American Indian older persons—have access to information about the availability of vision rehabilitation services (see Module 6).

Educational efforts need to include both the general public and professionals across many disciplines. They also need to target people in decision-making positions, including legislators and other policymakers, funders in the public and private arenas, and service planners, such as those in the aging network at the federal, state, and local levels.

5.2 Access to Vision Rehabilitation Services

To help older individuals obtain the vision services they need, both family members and the professionals who work with them need to have an understanding of both the types of services available (explained in Module 4) and the process for obtaining them, which is described in the following sections.

5.2.1 Eligibility for Vision-Related Rehabilitation Services

Eligibility for vision-related rehabilitation services has traditionally been determined by degree of vision loss. Each state has its own criteria for determining eligibility for vision rehabilitation services.

Typically, an individual must be designated as legally blind to be eligible for services, particularly for vocational rehabilitation (see Module 4). *Legal blindness* is defined as a visual acuity of no better than 20/200 in the better eye with the best possible correction, or a visual field of no more than 20 degrees (see the Glossary and Module 2 for a more detailed explanation).

However, in other instances, eligibility for services is determined by a classification of *severely visually impaired,* defined as having difficulty carrying out activities of daily living independently. This designation includes a larger number of individuals, particularly older persons who experience a serious loss of functional vision but do not meet the definition of legal blindness. It is also a more functional definition, determined by the degree of difficulty that results from the individual's level of vision loss (this term is discussed in more detail in Modules 1 and 2).

5.2.2 Obtaining Services

For the older person who is experiencing problems with vision, the eye care professional (an ophthalmologist or optometrist) is usually the first point of contact. In many cases, however, an individual contacts a vision rehabilitation agency first, and the agency suggests that the individual see an eye professional and inquire about a low vision evaluation. (Sources of referrals to eye care professionals include the American Academy of Ophthalmology and the American Optometric Association; see the Resources at the end of this module.)

The eye care professional is responsible for completing an eye report indicating an individual's degree of vision loss and, therefore, eligibility for vision rehabilitation services. The eye care professional sends the eye report to the state agency that oversees services for people who are blind or visually impaired—either a separate state agency serving individuals who are blind or visually impaired or a division or department for vision-related services within a general state vocational rehabilitation agency. This agency documents the individual's eligibility for services, opens the case, provides a case number, and assigns the case to a vision rehabilitation professional.

In some states, vision rehabilitation services are provided directly by the state rehabilitation agency. More frequently, the state rehabilitation agency contracts out to private, nonprofit vision rehabilitation agencies that provide the services to older consumers who are blind or visually impaired.

Typically, a caseworker or rehabilitation teacher is assigned the case and goes to the older person's home to conduct an assessment. Together, the rehabilitation teacher and the older person who is blind or visually impaired determine the type of assistance needed, the adaptive skills that the consumer needs to carry out routine daily tasks, and what the older person wants to be able to do independently. The specific skills taught by the rehabilitation teacher, the orientation and mobility (O&M) specialist, and the low vision instructor are described in detail in Module 4.

Vision rehabilitation services may be provided either in the older person's home or at a community-based agency offering individual or group instruction with other older visually impaired persons, or both. Agencies provide services in different ways, and these vary from community to community.

While the older visually impaired person is receiving vision rehabilitation services, a service provider in the aging network makes sure that needed support services are offered, such as Meals on Wheels, chore services, and escort services. Once the older visually impaired person acquires new adaptive skills, he or she may no longer need these services, depending on the individual's capacity to function independently.

During or after vision rehabilitation, older visually impaired persons may want to continue or resume participation in community activities, such as attending a senior center, or they may want to find new opportunities to be productive, such as volunteer work.

5.2.3 Effective Referrals

Understanding how the service delivery system works and the kinds of skills that an older person who is visually impaired may acquire can enable service providers in the aging field to understand how older visually impaired persons can continue to be active, contributing members of the community.

Rehabilitation services related to visual impairment can have the same positive impact of restoring functioning for the older blind or visually impaired person as physical and occupational therapies can have on those who experience physical dysfunctions as a result of injuries or stroke. Yet, many service providers are unfamiliar with these vision rehabilitation services and their eligibility criteria. Service providers in the aging field can have a positive impact on the lives of older persons who are losing their vision by making appropriate referrals and by following through to agencies that serve people who are blind or visually impaired.

When a service provider encounters an older person who is blind or visually impaired who is having difficulty functioning, the provider can initiate the following steps:

- Make sure the older person has seen an eye care professional, either an ophthalmologist or optometrist, and knows about his or

her visual acuity and eye condition. The individual's primary care physician can refer him or her to an eye care professional (see Resources for other sources of referrals).
- Ask if the older person has had a low vision evaluation and if he or she has received any instruction from an agency serving people who are blind or visually impaired. If not, encourage the older person to seek these services.

Some agencies that provide vision rehabilitation services also operate a low vision clinic on site or can make referrals to a low vision center. The *AFB Directory of Services for Blind and Visually Impaired Persons in the United States and Canada* (1997) provides a state-by-state listing of low vision centers and clinics.

The best strategy for service providers outside the vision field in making effective referrals to a low vision specialist is to get to know a key staff person at a local agency that serves older persons who are blind or visually impaired and establish a working relationship for effective mutual referrals.

5.2.4 Follow-Up and Follow-Through

Once a service provider has made a referral to an agency in the vision field, he or she cannot assume that the referral function is complete. To help avoid the common pitfalls of referrals, the service provider needs to make it routine to follow up to make sure that the consumer will be served by the vision agency and follow through to ensure that services are received. It is important, therefore, to determine the identity of the case manager at the agency to facilitate further contact.

Although the amount of time between referral, initial contact with the older person, and the beginning of rehabilitation services varies from state to state and community to community, many older persons experience a wait for rehabilitation because of the increased demand for services by the growing older population. When waiting lists are long, service providers need to maintain contact with potential clients. Older consumers can become discouraged by having to wait for services to start, especially if it took them a long time to make the decision to seek services.

Some services can begin while the newly visually impaired consumer is waiting for rehabilitation teaching services. These services may include Meals on Wheels, chore services, the provision of a senior companion, or telephone reassurance.

Perhaps the best example of a service agencies can offer to new clients while they are waiting for vision rehabilitation services to start is a support group. Joining a support group enables the older person to meet others experiencing similar reactions and difficulties in carrying out basic tasks, and from other older people they can learn ways to cope in the interim. (To find a local support group for newly visually impaired older persons, consult the Lighthouse *Directory of Self-Help/Mutual Aid Support Groups for Older People with Impaired Vision* [1994] or contact the Lighthouse National Center for Vision and Aging; see Resources.)

Once an individual begins to receive independent living skills training, he or she may continue to need supportive services from the aging network. If not, follow-through is still needed to ensure that after completion of vision rehabilitation services the older visually impaired person is reconnected to services and resources in the community for older persons.

It is likely that older visually impaired persons will not receive the vision rehabilitation services they need unless they and their family members, service providers in the aging network, and eye care professionals have access to information about available vision-related rehabilitation services. It is crucial, therefore, that older visually impaired consumers and their family members receive both adequate information, so that they can make informed decisions about services, and advocacy skills training, so that they feel empowered to be able to assertively seek services to which they are entitled.

Participants in advocacy skills training can learn how to make sure they get the information they need from busy service providers such as physicians, how to be assertive about stating their needs, how to ask the right questions, and so on. This training should be included as part of the package of vision rehabilitation services for adults of all ages, but especially for older persons. The availability of advocacy skills training programs for older consumers is still quite limited, and this is an area that both the aging and vision rehabilitation fields need to address (see Module 6).

5.3 Home- and Community-Based Long-Term Services

When older persons are told that they have an eye condition associated with gradually deteriorating vision, their first thoughts are frequently, "Will I be able to continue to take care of myself and continue to live in my own home, or will I need to go to a nursing home?" Family members experience similar fears that their relative will no longer be able to live independently and that nursing home placement may be the best or the only option.

In a majority of cases, however, placing the person in a nursing home would be premature, unnecessary, costly to the individual and family members, and not cost-effective for the service delivery system. For most older people, particularly those for whom vision loss is the only factor threatening their independent functioning, in-home and community-based services can enable them to continue to live independently with or without the assistance of others. This assistance can come from family members and neighbors as well as from professionals in the aging and vision rehabilitation fields.

The term home- and community-based care (HCBC) refers to programs that offer the full range of services and settings available to elderly or disabled people to enable them to continue living either in their own homes or in a residential care setting.

The basic community services available through an HCBC system include the following:

- information and assistance
- personal care, homemaker, and chore services
- congregate and home-delivered meals
- adult day care
- rehabilitative care
- transportation assistance
- home health care
- caregivers' support, assistance, and respite care
- housing options, including assisted-living arrangements
- consumer protection and advocacy

Because many older people and individuals with disabilities have multiple and changing health and social service needs, effective HCBC programs can facilitate access to, and networking among, the basic services provided by offering "one-stop-shopping" arrangements, comprehensive assessment, care planning or case management, pre–nursing home admission screening, and linkage to medical care providers.

As the aging of the baby boomers proceeds, the number of elderly people requiring long-term care will also grow. States and localities, all of whom have a major financial stake in containing Medicaid costs, are increasingly looking toward HCBC as a possible alternative for reducing the growth of long-term care expenditures. And, because older people and people with disabilities want to remain in their own homes and communities for as long as possible, rather than in institutions, the demand for such comprehensive care will continue to rise as well. This growing need has major implications for caregiving, as well as for employment and health care policies.

5.3.1 The Aging Network and HCBC

The aging network strives to provide a full range of HCBC services and administrative systems to meet the needs of older people and people with disabilities and their caregivers in every region and community across the country.

The network's 57 State Units on Aging (SUAs), 655 Area Agencies on Aging (AAAs), 222 tribal organizations representing 300 Native American tribes, and thousands of service providers plan, advocate for, coordinate, and develop services for the elderly. The aging network is in a strategic position to use its long-standing experience and expertise to meet the needs of older persons for long-term care.

As a critical function of administering Older Americans Act funds, many SUAs and AAAs have coordinated multiple sources of funds for long-term care, including the administration of the Medicaid Home- and Community-Based Waiver and Personal Care Option Programs, the most flexible source of funds for HCBC. Many AAAs fund the delivery of basic HCBC services by local service providers to deliver basic HCBC services through state allocations of Older Americans Act funds, state and local revenues, Social Services Block Grant funds, and other resources. AAAs also are extensively involved in case management services to ensure that older persons are linked to the services they need. Information on the SUAs as well as the provider of independent living programs in each state can be found in the *AFB Directory of Services* (1997). In addition, the Eldercare Locator, operated by the Administration on Aging, provides the name and telephone number of the nearest AAA (see the Resources at the end of this module).

At present, there are approximately 2 million Americans living in long-term care institutions such as nursing homes and other adult care settings (*Profile of Older Americans,* 1997). By comparison, more than 10 million persons of all ages need some type of assistance with their activities of daily living in order to remain in their own homes or in other community-based settings. Approximately 45 percent of persons requiring home- and community-based care are between the ages of 18 and 65, and much of the remaining 55 percent are over the age of 65.

5.3.2 Vision Rehabilitation and HCBC

Home- and community-based long-term services are essential resources for older people who are blind or severely visually impaired. The ongoing supportive services these programs provide can improve the quality of life for individuals who are blind or severely visually impaired and can enable them to continue to be contributing members of their families and communities (Lidoff, 1995, 1996).

Two-thirds of older persons who are severely visually impaired also have at least one other serious disability or chronic illness. Such individuals may already receive home- and community-based services, but they may need additional services and special accommodations related to their vision loss.

Thus, the inclusion of vision-related rehabilitation in a long-term services package would help restore the independence of people who are severely visually impaired and reduce their need for ongoing supportive services (Lidoff, 1995). (Inclusion of vision services in HCBC programs is discussed in more detail in Module 6.) Rehabilitation that assists visually impaired individuals to comply with medical regimens, manage their medications, and avoid injuries would also sustain their independence and help contain health care costs.

However, eligibility requirements for HCBC programs may make it difficult for some older people who are blind or visually impaired to receive these services. For example, an older person whose only impairment is severe vision loss might not qualify for a program whose eligibility is limited to people who are unable to perform certain basic activities of daily living (ADLs), such as eating, bathing, dressing, using the bathroom, and transferring in and out of bed. Yet, such a person might be unable to perform the cluster of instrumental activities of daily living (IADLs) that comprise each of the basic ADLs.

For instance, although an individual may be able to eat, he or she may be unable to get to the market, select the proper foods, or prepare food safely in the kitchen. Similarly, an individual may be able to get in and out of bed but may not be able to maintain proper orientation and balance or to move around safely inside the home or outdoors (Lidoff, 1995).

People with severe vision loss also are likely to have difficulty handling finances and taking medications, two IADLs that, in and of themselves, have a major impact on the ability to live independently.

Vision-related rehabilitation, with its goal of promoting independent living and a high quality of life, is a natural component of home- and community-based services. The choice of services and assistive devices needs to be based on an assessment of a person's functional capacity and individual needs.

5.3.3 Improving Access to HCBC Services

Professionals in the aging network who administer home- and community-based long-term care programs can facilitate access to these services for older people who are blind or severely visually impaired by being aware of their needs when they conduct outreach, communicate with and assess clients, and provide services. A number of strategies can help these service providers be more responsive to the needs of older people who are blind or visually impaired (Lidoff, 1995).

Organizations conducting outreach strategies need to consider the following strategies:

- Provide the state rehabilitation agency serving people who are blind or visually impaired with information about available home- and community-based long-term services.
- Use radio and television, in addition to newspapers, for public service announcements. Publicize home- and community-based long-term services programs on community radio reading services, which are designed for use by people who have difficulty reading regular print.
- Ask usual referral sources such as physicians, senior programs, churches and synagogues, and other groups to be on the lookout for people who may be experiencing vision loss. People who are visually impaired may be socially isolated.

The following strategies will be helpful in effective communication with clients:

- Make program materials available in large print, at least 18-point type.
- Offer clients assistance with reading forms and transportation to appointments.
- When talking, face clients and speak directly to them, since many older people with vision loss also have a hearing impairment. Always let a person who is visually impaired know if you are moving away or leaving the room.

It is important to include questions related to visual functioning in assessment instruments. Ask assessment questions that are sufficiently sensitive to identify specific functional problems resulting from vision loss. For example:

- Can you see to read the newspaper?
- Can you read your mail?
- Can you read labels on medicine bottles?
- Can you read street signs?
- Can you recognize faces of family or friends across a room?

Agencies in the aging network can use the following strategies in the provision of services:

- Learn about the services and eligibility requirements of public and private agencies for people who are blind and visually impaired.
- Ask such agencies to provide in-service training for staff who work in intake, care management, and direct service to help them learn to recognize signs of vision loss, communicate effectively with people who are visually impaired, and make appropriate service contracts and referrals.
- Consider making individual counseling and support groups available for both people with recent vision loss and family members or other informal caregivers to help in adjusting to this major life change.
- Remember that once people have received vision rehabilitation services and have learned to cope with a vision loss, they still may have ongoing needs for assistance such as readers and drivers (Lidoff, 1995).

5.4 Access to Services in Nursing Homes

Notwithstanding the range of supportive and long-term care services available in the community, placement in a nursing home can sometimes be the best option for an older individual who requires a level of care that cannot be provided through home- and community-based care and by family members. However, vision loss alone should not be the criterion for nursing home placement. Most older people with impaired vision in long-term care facilities have additional health problems or physical impairments that made nursing home placement necessary.

Nursing home placement is an appropriate option for some older people only after other in-home or community-based options have been explored. In fact, the best predictor of nursing home placement is usually the limited availability or lack of family members or other in-home caregivers.

Older people who are blind or visually impaired and live in nursing homes may benefit from the services of rehabilitation teachers and O&M specialists, just as they would if they were living in the community. However, many such residents do not have access to independent living skills and environmental orientation training that would enable them to function as independently as possible while in the nursing home. Limited access to these services is most frequently the result of the fact that nursing home staff do not know about vision rehabilitation services for this population.

In addition, with the limited funds available to provide older persons with the independent living skills they need, priority must by necessity be given to those individuals who will be able to continue to live at home as a result of these services. Therefore, even if called upon, a vision rehabilitation agency may only be able to provide in-service training to the nursing home staff, unless the agency has other funds with which to provide rehabilitation services.

In-service training available from local agencies that serve people who are blind or visually impaired can be helpful for nursing home staff at all levels, from administrators to maintenance workers, to assist them in understanding the services that visually impaired residents of their facilities may require. (See the Resources for curricula on working with residents who are blind or visually impaired in long-term care settings.)

5.5 An Eye Toward the Future

As future generations of individuals reach age 55 and older and experience age-related vision loss, much more will need to be done to increase the level of awareness about their concerns and needs to make sure that these issues are addressed and services are provided.

For example, as older people who are severely visually impaired become more visible as active, productive, and contributing members of their communities, their family members, service providers, the general public, and older people themselves will recognize and acknowledge the importance of making this group a priority in public policy and services.

Members of the baby boom generation, many of whom are family caregivers now, are finding out about existing resources. Consequently, they will become a very different generation when they reach their own senior years. They will know more about the services that exist, the eligibility criteria, and how to gain access to the service system. They will know that rehabilitation services are not just for the young or for those of working age (as traditionally conceived), and they will understand the benefits of independent living skills training.

Children today are increasingly aware of and comfortable with other children with disabilities who are becoming a visible part of mainstream education and community life. They are therefore also in a better position to understand, as they grow up, that older people also need to be part of the mainstream of community life.

Blindness has traditionally been designated as a low-incidence disability compared to other disabilities, but with the dramatic demographic shift in the population of individuals who are blind or severely visually impaired this is no longer the case. This perception must change at the policy and service delivery levels so that vision-related services get the attention, priority, and funding they deserve.

Losing one's vision does not have to mean losing one's way of life. Vision loss should not mean forced early retirement, but it can if the individual and the employer do not know where to turn for help or even that help is available. The Title VII, Chapter 2 independent living program needs a broader base of supporters and advocates beyond the leadership of the vision field. Older people themselves, their family members, and professionals outside the vision field have to educate their legislators about the need for the Chapter 2 program, the number of people it reaches, and its cost-effectiveness.

Practitioners in the vision field are taking a closer look at the outcomes of vision-related rehabilitation services to be in the best position to make clear to key decision makers that vision rehabilitation services can make a significant difference to the independent functioning and quality of life for older people who experience age-related vision loss. Module 6 examines this trend in greater detail, along with other changes in the field that are enabling older individuals to gain greater access to the vision rehabilitation and related services they need.

References

AFB directory of services for blind and visually impaired persons in the United States and Canada (25th ed.). (1997). New York: AFB Press.

A directory of self-help/mutual aid support groups for older people with impaired vision. (1994). New York: The Lighthouse.

Biegel, D. E., Petchers, M. K., Snyder, A., & Beisgin, B. (1989). Unmet needs and barriers to service delivery for the blind and visually impaired elderly. *Gerontologist, 29*(1), 86–91.

Lidoff, L. (1995). Home- and community-based long-term services: A resource for adults who are visually impaired. *Journal of Visual Impairment & Blindness, 89*(6), 541–545.

Lidoff, L. (1996). Home- and community-based long-term services: Action steps. *Journal of Visual Impairment & Blindness, 90*(4), 15–16.

Lidoff, L. (1997). Moving vision-related rehabilitation into the U.S. health care mainstream. *Journal of Visual Impairment & Blindness, 91*(2), 107–116.

Massof, R. W. (1996). Low vision rehabilitation in the U.S. health care system. *Journal of Vision Rehabilitation, 9*(3), 1–31.

National Advisory Eye Council. (1993). *Vision research: A national plan, 1994–1998.* Bethesda, MD: National Eye Institute, National Institutes of Health.

Profile of older Americans: 1997. (1997). Washington, DC: American Association of Retired Persons, Program Resources Department, and Administration on Aging, U.S. Department of Health and Human Services.

Stuen, C. (1991). Awareness of resources for visually impaired older adults among the aging network. In N. Weber (Ed.), *Vision and aging: Issues in social work practice.* New York: Haworth University Press.

RECOMMENDED TEACHING METHODS

Lecture or Guest Speaker

Describe the eligibility criteria for vision rehabilitation services, the referral process, and the importance of follow-up from the aging network or invite a guest speaker from a local office of the state rehabilitation area to address students on these topics.

Small-Group Brainstorming

Organize students into small groups of four or five, and have the groups identify the possible barriers that the family in the following scenario may experience when trying to get the grandmother to accept vision-related services:

> Mrs. A., a grandmother living with her grown daughter Rosa and her family, grew up and raised her children in Puerto Rico until they were in their teens. Mrs. A has been experiencing increasing difficulty seeing to read, getting around the house, cooking, and doing other household chores. The grandmother maintains that she is fine, and that this is just what happens as you get older.

Role Playing

Present a scenario in which a family visits an agency for elderly persons, seeking services for an older family member who is losing vision. Ask students to role play the referral process, expressing the client's needs and the family's interest in being involved.

Have students go through the actual steps of identifying resources and gathering information firsthand about how to gain access to services for clients.

RESOURCES

Recommended Readings

Griffin-Shirley, N., & Groff, G. (1993). *Prescriptions for independence: Working with older people who are visually impaired.* New York: American Foundation for the Blind.

Horowitz, A. (1994). Vision impairment and functional disability among nursing home residents. *The Gerontologist, 34*(3), 316–323.

Horowitz, A., Balistreri, E., Stuen, C., & Fangmeier, R. (1995). Vision status and rehabilitation needs among nursing home residents. *Journal of Visual Impairment & Blindness, 89*(1), 7–15.

Orr, A. L. (1993). American Indian elders: Diabetes, diabetic retinopathy and the need for independent living skills training. *Journal of Visual Impairment & Blindness, 97*(9), 336–341.

Orr, A. L. (1994). Improving access to services for older visually impaired persons: Executive summary. In A. L. Orr, L. Lidoff, & J. Scott (Eds.), *Building bridges: A resource packet for serving older visually impaired persons.* New York: American Foundation for the Blind.

Further Readings

Beach, J. D., Robinet, J. M., & Hakim-Larson, J. (1995). Self-esteem and independent living skills of adults with visual impairments. *Journal of Visual Impairment & Blindness, 89*(6), 531–540.

Hersen, M., Kabacoff, R. I., Van Hasselt, V. B., Null, J. A., Ryan, C. F., Melton, M. A., & Segal, D. L. (1995). Assertiveness, depression and social support in older visually impaired adults. *Journal of Visual Impairment & Blindness, 89*(6), 524–530.

Horowitz, A., & Balistreri, E. (1994). *Field initiated research to evaluate methods for the identification and treatment of visually impaired nursing home residents.* New York: The Lighthouse.

Other Materials

A directory of self-help/mutual aid support groups for older people with impaired vision. (1994). New York: The Lighthouse.

A directory containing state-by-state listings of over 670 support groups, plus self-help clearinghouses, state agencies for the blind and visually impaired, private vision rehabilitation agencies that work with older people, national resource organizations, and a bibliography of books and articles on organizing and facilitating support groups.

Duffy, M., & Beliveau-Toby, M. (1992). *New independence for older persons with vision loss in long-term care facilities.* Mohegan Lake, NY: AWARE.

A three-part training kit that presents a multidisciplinary team approach to problem solving, with the older visually impaired person as the center of the team. The kit includes a learner workbook, facilitator's guide, resource manual, and vision simulators.

Fangmeier, R. (1994). *The World Through Their Eyes.* New York: The Lighthouse.
A 21-minute videotape and manual for training nursing home staff that identifies concerns of older people who are visually impaired and illustrates strategies for care in residential health care settings.

Organizations

The organizations listed here include those that are working at a national level to improve the integration between the aging and vision service delivery systems. Also listed here are sources of referrals for eye care services. Additional sources of information and referral are listed in the Resources to Module 2.

Administration on Aging
U.S. Department of Health and Human Services
200 Independence Avenue, S.W.
Washington, DC 20201
(202) 401-4634 or (800) 677-1116 (Eldercare Locator)
http://www.aoa.dhhs.gov

Acts as an advocate for the elderly within the federal government. Administers the Older Americans Act of 1965 to assist states and local communities in developing comprehensive service systems for older persons. Operates the Eldercare Locator, a national toll-free information and assistance directory, at (800) 677-1116, for older people and caregivers, which provides the name and telephone number of the nearest Area Agency on Aging.

American Academy of Ophthalmology
P.O. Box 7424
San Francisco, CA 94120-7424
(800) 222-EYES (helpline)
http://www.aao.org

Sponsors the National Eye Care Project, whose helpline number refers callers to local ophthalmologists who will provide free eye care to older people in need. State affiliates can also provide referrals.

American Optometric Association
243 North Lindbergh Boulevard
St. Louis, MO 63141
(314) 991-4100 or (800) 262-2210

FAX: (314) 991-4101
http://www.aoanet.org

Provides free consumer information materials on eye health and vision. Has a low vision section that provides consumer information and referrals.

Lighthouse National Center for Vision and Aging
11 East 59th Street
New York, NY 10022
(212) 821-9200 or (800) 334-5497 or TDD (212) 821-9713
FAX: (212) 821-9705
http://www.lighthouse.org

Serves as a national clearinghouse for information on vision and aging and referrals to services.

National Association of Area Agencies on Aging
1112 16th Street, N.W., Suite 100
Washington, DC 20036
(202) 296-8130
FAX: (202) 296-8134
E-mail: jjfn4a@erols.com

Provides referrals to local Area Agencies on Aging.

National Association of State Units on Aging
1225 I Street, N.W., Suite 725
Washington, DC 20005
(202) 898-2578
FAX: (202) 898-2583
E-mail: staff@nasua.org

Provides information on state services to older persons and advocates for legislation and funding for such services.

National Council of State Agencies for the Blind
1213 29th Street, N.W.
Washington, DC 20007
(202) 298-8468
FAX: (202) 333-5881

Promotes communication among agencies involved in preventing blindness and offering services to individuals who are severely visually impaired.

MODULE 6

Trends and Issues in Vision-Related Rehabilitation Services

This module discusses the need to develop new services and new components of service delivery models. It gives an overview of current trends in the delivery of vision-related rehabilitation services, including the use of family rehabilitation models, community-based satellite sites, and peers in mentorship and leadership models; as well as the emphasis on social integration and mainstreaming, empowerment and advocacy skills training programs, outreach services, and opportunities for productive activity such as volunteerism and mentoring. This module also explores current issues in the vision rehabilitation field, including the need for increased funding and diversified funding sources, for the preservation of specialized services for people who are blind or visually impaired, and for advocacy to influence public policy. Finally, the module discusses the future of service delivery.

Topic Outline

6.1 Current Trends in the Delivery of Vision-Related Rehabilitation Services

    6.1.1 The Family Rehabilitation Model

    6.1.2 Community-Based Satellite Sites

    6.1.3 The Role of Peers in Vision Rehabilitation

6.1.4 The Provision of Mental Health Services

6.1.5 Social Integration and Mainstreaming

6.1.6 Empowerment and Advocacy Skills Training Programs

6.1.7 Outreach Services: Methods for Identifying Hard-to-Reach Populations

6.1.8 Opportunities for Successful Aging and Productive Activity

6.1.9 Collaborative Models

6.2 Current Issues in the Vision Rehabilitation Field

6.2.1 Funding Issues

6.2.2 Vision Rehabilitation Therapists

6.2.3 Specialized Vision-Related Services

6.2.4 Public Policy

6.3 The Future of Service Delivery

Learner Objectives

1. The student will be able to describe current trends in the delivery of vision-related rehabilitation services to older people who are blind or visually impaired.

2. The student will be able to identify innovative services and models of service delivery that are helping agencies that serve older people who are blind or visually impaired meet the needs of this population.

3. The student will be able to describe current issues in the vision rehabilitation field, including the need for increased and diversified funding, restorative therapeutic intervention, and the need to preserve specialized vision-related services.

6.1 Current Trends in the Delivery of Vision-Related Rehabilitation Services

As a result of the continuing growth in the population of older people who are blind or visually impaired, vision rehabilitation is a growing and changing field. This module discusses current trends and issues in delivering vision-related rehabilitation services.

Many people view "the elderly" as a monolithic group whose needs can be addressed with one set of solutions. However, as noted in Module 1, this population can be viewed as consisting of four age cohorts: ages 55–64, 65–74, 75–84, and 85 and older. When these cohorts are examined separately, it can be seen that each one consists of individuals with differing degrees of physical, psychological, and cognitive functioning and an equally diverse range of interests, abilities, and desires for activity and independent functioning.

Agencies have taken on this challenge by developing additional service components to supplement core services, as well as new methods of delivering services to meet the needs of an increasingly diverse population of older persons. Agencies that recognize the need for such innovation first take an inventory of their resources and of the population needing service, make a strategic plan for a creative means of enhancing their ongoing services, and then implement the plan incrementally as resources (funding, personnel, volunteers, and such) are available and can be used creatively for maximum results.

In many cases, the innovations that have been instituted in vision rehabilitation are unique to the field; in other instances, they have been borrowed from disciplines that serve other special populations. Among these innovative services or service delivery methods are the following:

- a focus on serving the family unit, using such models as family rehabilitation and caregiver support groups
- provision of services in satellite sites in the community
- the use of peers in mentorship and leadership models
- provision of mental health services
- self-help and mutual-aid support groups
- social integration and mainstreaming strategies
- empowerment and advocacy skills training programs
- innovative community outreach strategies to identify hard-to-reach populations and improve access for older consumers
- programs that create opportunities for productive activity through volunteerism and employment opportunities
- collaborative models with the aging network and other related fields and disciplines

Vision-related rehabilitation services or therapies are part of the continuum of home- and community-based long-term care services

MODULE 6: TRENDS AND ISSUES IN VISION-RELATED REHABILITATION SERVICES

(see Module 5). Like physical, occupational, and speech therapies, vision-related services enable older persons to continue to live as independently as possible within their own homes and communities, avoiding premature and unnecessary nursing home placements.

Yet, in this era of scarce resources, agencies that serve people who are blind or visually impaired face severe limitations in essential resources such as funding and personnel, just when substantial changes are needed to serve the growing number of older people in need along with the traditional population of younger clients.

This situation constitutes a challenge to agencies to be creative rather than be burdened by the limitations: to move beyond the confines of the agency and the field and to maximize the resources and expertise of the community and related service fields. The innovative services and methods of service delivery that are described in the following sections illustrate ways in which agencies are already meeting this challenge.

These innovative services represent components of a comprehensive model of service to older persons that views and serves the older person holistically. Although the innovations discussed in the following sections are presented as separate service components, there is considerable overlap in benefits to consumers and in the overall goals of vision-related rehabilitation and self-actualization.

6.1.1 The Family Rehabilitation Model

The family rehabilitation model has become very important in ensuring successful integration of independent living skills for older people and for their family members as well. In this model, one or more family members are an active part of the vision rehabilitation process.

The family rehabilitation model strives to include and encourage the involvement of significant others during independent living skills training and orientation and mobility (O&M) instruction. Such involvement benefits the family members as well as the newly visually impaired person. Family members understand that their relative can learn techniques to be safe and confident, and they can learn the adaptive skills along with their older relative. Through this involvement, family members support the visually impaired individual while helping to reinforce the skills taught by service providers.

In a recent study, the anxiety level of family members was greatly reduced by the knowledge that their elderly relative had been taught independent living skills (Crews & Frey, 1993).

The family rehabilitation model also has benefits after the provision of vision rehabilitation services: Family members are able to reinforce the adaptive techniques if the older individual needs follow-up assistance.

6.1.2   Community-Based Satellite Sites

Another rehabilitation innovation is the provision of services at satellite sites of the agency, most commonly a senior center or other community facility, where rehabilitation teachers instruct older consumers in independent living skills.

This method eliminates the need for the consumer to come to an agency "for the blind," a label that many older people view as stigmatizing. The added benefit is that the individual is able either to continue to use a familiar community resource in the aging network or to be introduced to an important new resource.

The staff of the center and senior citizens with normal vision also benefit from learning more about the services offered by agencies that serve blind and visually impaired persons and about the abilities of their visually impaired peers. Instruction in this everyday environment also facilitates the social integration of visually impaired individuals as well as the identification of new clients and referrals.

6.1.3   The Role of Peers in Vision Rehabilitation

A number of innovative rehabilitation strategies are based on the use of peers—other older individuals who are visually impaired—to assist in providing services.

Peer Instruction

Agencies are training older visually impaired persons who have already received rehabilitation training to teach independent living skills to their peers under the supervision of a rehabilitation professional. Peer instruction is a valuable strategy in many ways.

Peer instruction is an effective way in which to empower people. It enhances the self-confidence and self-esteem of the instructor who is demonstrating his or her newly acquired skills and performing a productive service. It also helps the peer instructors' clients as they learn from a high-functioning, motivated role model who resembles themselves. An additional benefit to the agency involved is that peer instructors help to ameliorate financial and personnel shortages in times of scarce resources.

Peer Counseling

Increasingly, agencies are training older persons who are blind or visually impaired, and who have recently completed vision rehabilitation, to serve as peer counselors. Many individuals feel more comfortable talking with a peer who has experienced, or is still experiencing, some of the same struggles they are confronting as a result of their loss of vision.

Peer Support Groups

Peer support groups are among the fastest-growing services provided to older people experiencing vision loss. Support groups offer an excellent opportunity for participants to get to know other individuals who are experiencing circumstances similar to their own. They learn from each other's experiences and strategies for coping, and they share solutions to common problems and difficulties. Support groups vary in the ways they are structured and run.

To find a local support group for newly visually impaired older persons, consult the Lighthouse *Directory of Self-Help/Mutual Aid Support Groups* (1994), or contact the Lighthouse National Center for Vision and Aging (see the Resources section at the end of this module.)

6.1.4 *The Provision of Mental Health Services*

Some older people who experience age-related vision loss may need more than a support group or peer counseling services to deal with the issues related to losing their vision. Various agencies that serve older people who are blind or visually impaired are making effective use of clinical social workers or clinical psychologists who can provide the expertise and environment necessary to ensure the psychological well-being of older individuals.

When it is not possible to have clinical specialists working on staff or as consultants, agencies that serve older people who are blind or visually impaired develop effective partnerships with local agencies in the fields of aging and mental health that provide mental health services. For example, one agency developed a project with a local mental health association to help older persons who are developmentally disabled and visually impaired make the transition from a facility-based employment setting (previously referred to as a sheltered workshop) to the senior center environment.

Professionals in the vision rehabilitation field continue to examine the possibilities of creating links with professionals in other fields, including mental health.

6.1.5 Social Integration and Mainstreaming

The concept of integrating or mainstreaming individuals with various functional limitations into ordinary environments has long been associated with the educational environment of children with disabilities. However, the same principles apply to the needs of older people who also want access to nonspecialized services, resources, and environments or would want it if they thought it was possible.

Senior centers can be a lifeline in combating social isolation for many older persons who are visually impaired. Thus, making sure that older visually impaired individuals have full access to senior centers can be an important strategy for this group.

A New York agency that recognized the need to integrate visually impaired persons into all aspects of senior center life developed a model with the following essential elements (Ludwig & Schneider, 1991):

- training center staff about the needs and capabilities of potential clients who are visually impaired
- providing sensitivity training about blindness and visual impairment for senior citizens who attend the center
- training visually impaired older individuals themselves before introducing them to a mainstream setting, in order to make them comfortable with the environment

Several agencies throughout the country have since adopted similar models of integration. Community integration is one of the seven designated categories of services under Title VII, Chapter 2 of the Rehabilitation Act—the Independent Living Services for Older Individuals Who Are Blind program (see Module 4). Many funded agencies have been working toward this goal since Chapter 2 funds were first available, but it is not yet a major trend.

Nevertheless, older people who are blind or visually impaired are still included in the senior center environment only on a limited basis. Considerable public and professional education is still needed at many levels to dispel negative and stereotypic thinking about the limitations of older people who are blind or visually impaired (see Module 5).

Agencies in the vision field are working with agencies in the field of aging to ensure that older blind or visually impaired individuals are included and integrated into programs for older people. For example, as already noted, agencies serving people who are blind or visually impaired make use of senior centers for a variety of purposes, including conducting support groups and assigning rehabilitation teachers to teach independent living skills and O&M instructors to teach O&M skills to members who are visually impaired.

Providing vision-related services in the senior center environment also allows other members of the center to become familiar with these services and to have easy access to them in the event they are needed. Many vision rehabilitation agencies also provide community education and in-service training to senior center staff and members about the needs and capabilities of older visually impaired persons and about the agency as a community service and resource.

Senior centers are essential community resources, and much more needs to be done to make maximum use of them. However, efforts toward integration can be staff intensive for both the senior center and the agency that serves blind and visually impaired persons. (See the fact sheet on "Integrating Older Persons Who Are Visually Impaired into a Senior Center or Other Community Activity" at the end of this module and "Tips for Adapting Leisure and Recreational Activities for Individuals Who Are Blind or Visually Impaired" in Module 4). A strong collaborative partnership between the two agencies and joint commitment are essential for success (see Module 7).

6.1.6 Empowerment and Advocacy Skills Training Programs

Many groups of individuals with disabilities have established an effective political voice to make their needs known and their abilities recognized, both within the community and on a national level. Individuals with physical disabilities, particularly those who use wheelchairs, have educated the general public about issues of accessibility. Individuals who are blind or visually impaired, including older persons, have not organized to as great an extent to establish an effective political voice.

Older persons often feel disempowered by their loss of vision and are sometimes unable to get the services they need to participate in many aspects of community life and activity. An important and yet often overlooked aspect of service delivery is teaching advocacy skills, including essential information, to older persons with disabilities in order to empower them—literally give them the power—to get their needs addressed. Service planners and providers in both the aging and the vision-related rehabilitation fields need increasingly to offer advocacy skills training.

Empowerment training is an effective and necessary strategy for enhancing feelings of self-efficacy—the individual's belief in his or her personal power to control his or her own life. Ensuring self-efficacy for the older person who is experiencing age-related vision loss is an important goal of vision rehabilitation.

Vision rehabilitation programs can also empower older individuals by their method of service delivery and attitude, and by establishing roles for peer trainers and peer counselors.

For example, some private agencies have developed their own approaches to introducing older persons to services and the service environment. One agency uses an innovative "explorer approach" to introduce older people to its array of available services. Potential clients are invited to visit the agency for a full day to see firsthand the kinds of services available to them. Two consumers are paired to go through the experience together, and each can determine the most appropriate services for himself or herself. Family members are also invited to participate. The explorer approach serves as a client-centered, client-driven approach to service, giving the client some control of the vision rehabilitation process and demonstrating to the client from the outset that he or she is an active participant in the decision about the type of skills training he or she will receive. It also serves as an innovative intake procedure.

The support-group environment and structure can also serve to empower newly visually impaired persons. Advocacy skills can be an important topic for one or more sessions of weekly support groups, particularly those that are ongoing.

Despite the importance of advocacy skills, many agencies serving visually impaired persons have not yet developed advocacy skills training programs to help their clients find ways to get their needs met beyond the environment of the vision rehabilitation agency. Some agencies have not recognized the need for this training. Those that have must be sure that their limited resources provide for the most essential core services first.

Service providers in the field of aging can be effective advocates for clients who are experiencing vision loss when they understand how the vision rehabilitation system operates.

6.1.7 Outreach Services: Methods for Identifying Hard-to-Reach Populations

Agencies serving older persons who are blind or visually impaired are faced with the challenge of identifying older persons who are not seeking services because they are not aware that the services exist or that they are eligible for these services. It is especially important for agencies to be attuned to the groups of people who may not be seeking services because of language or cultural barriers, or those who have limited access to services as a result of geographic or income-level barriers within the service area (see Module 5).

It is a mistake to assume that because members of minority groups are not seeking out services, the need for services does not exist or that these older persons are being taken care of within their nuclear or extended family units. Agencies need effective outreach strategies to reach minority groups, particularly older African-American, Hispanic, and American Indian persons, whose incidence of blindness and visual impairment is documented to be higher than the average rate among Caucasian Americans (see Module 1). Many people in Asian communities also are responsive to bicultural outreach but would not otherwise seek services. It is equally important to be aware of the rise in new immigrant populations such as Russian, Haitian, and other refugee groups, who are also in need of vision-related rehabilitation services.

The most effective outreach is often carried out by bilingual and bicultural personnel—professional or paraprofessional staff or volunteers—who are in the best position to understand which strategies are successful in reaching a specific population and can carry out educational efforts in the language of the community. It is also important to train minority-group members as paraprofessionals to minimize language and cultural barriers to service.

Because members of minority groups are not at present sufficiently represented as professionals in the field of vision rehabilitation, strategic recruitment of minority-group members into rehabilitation teaching and O&M instruction has been a priority for many years. University programs in these disciplines also conduct outreach to members of minority groups. This is an issue that requires continued attention.

Agencies need to continue to develop bilingual and bicultural outreach and service delivery in order to help ensure that they are serving the entire population within their service area.

6.1.8 Opportunities for Successful Aging and Productive Activity

Productive or successful aging is an important concept in the field of aging. The word "productive" has traditionally been associated with remunerative employment. But when applied in gerontology, it is intended to mean much more. Productive aging for any older person, including one who is blind or visually impaired, can include any of the following:

- being gainfully employed
- providing volunteer service to others
- making contributions to the community through involvement with and leadership in community organizations
- serving as a mentor or role model for others, particularly other people with disabilities or children
- continuing to assume active roles within the family and social context
- caring for others as a family or neighboring caregiver

For older individuals, caring for oneself, functioning independently, and maintaining existing social roles are also productive activities.

Many older persons who experience age-related vision loss assume, at least initially, that they are no longer able to be productive or contributing members in their family, the community, the workforce, or other areas in which they have had significant and valued roles and responsibilities.

Many professionals and service providers who come in contact with older visually impaired persons are likewise unaware of their potential to make contributions after the onset of vision loss. Yet awareness of this potential is critical for these professionals to be able to inspire, encourage, and provide a vision of competence and continued functioning to older persons experiencing age-related vision loss.

Paid Employment

Many older persons who experience the onset of visual impairment while they are still employed want to continue to work. This is particularly true of people who are still under the traditional retirement age of 65 or 70. And as the life span increases, many older individuals are preferring to remain employed longer. Yet because many older visually impaired persons perceive themselves as having no employment potential, they allow themselves to be forced into premature retirement.

Through the use of adaptive technology, assistive devices, and adaptive skills training, many such individuals can continue in their jobs as they were or with slight modifications. But opportunities need to be broadened.

Employers and human resource personnel need to be educated to recognize that older individuals with impaired vision (like individuals of all ages with impaired vision) can be productive and contributing members of the work force. For example, a vocational counselor can work with an employer and employee to understand the essential parts of jobs and how job sharing and job modification could be used to help the individual with a disability remain in the workforce. These forms of accommodation involve modifying a job's nonessential tasks to suit the best abilities of an individual with a disability, or allowing a co-worker to assist an individual with certain aspects of a job that are difficult to perform because of the individual's disability.

In addition to employers, service providers and older people themselves need to recognize and respond to the capacity for employment of older visually impaired persons.

Some agencies have begun to make employment-related services a priority for older persons. Older people experiencing age-related vision loss need easier and greater access to vocational rehabilitation services including vocational rehabilitation counseling (Moore,

Graves, & Patterson, 1997) so that they can remain in or reenter the job market. It is much easier to help a capable individual who is visually impaired to remain in the workforce than to help the same person reenter the job market. Early intervention and self-advocacy on the part of the older individual are both essential. When such services are accessible, older visually impaired persons can be employed in either competitive or supported employment.

Whichever type of employment opportunity is possible, returning to a previous job or a career or beginning a newly created job provides the older worker who is visually impaired with a valued role and a new social network at a critical stage of the life cycle.

Agencies also need to consider developing employer-training programs to educate human resource personnel about the potential of older people who are visually impaired as reliable, competent employees.

Another relatively untapped resource for employment for older individuals who are visually impaired is Title V of the federal Older Americans Act, which created the Senior Community Service Employment Program for Older Americans. This program provides employment, primarily in human service organizations, for low-income older persons. Agencies in the vision field may want to consider developing a cooperative relationship with their local Area Agency on Aging—the agency designated by the federal Administration on Aging to develop and coordinate services for the elderly (see Module 5)—to create work opportunities in the community. A human service organization can be a supportive working environment for an older person who is visually impaired and who wishes to reenter the job market.

Planning for the 21st century requires planning for a changing labor force and for greater job and workplace flexibility to accommodate an older, more experienced labor force. Members of the baby boom generation will need to continue working beyond the traditional retirement age to support older parents. Early retirement should be a choice, not a requirement, for older Americans, including those experiencing vision loss and other disabilities.

Opportunities for Volunteer Service

Many older persons, including those with vision problems, may prefer retirement to employment. Even so, a large number of them will

MODULE 6:
TRENDS AND ISSUES
IN VISION-RELATED
REHABILITATION
SERVICES

want to find new outlets for creative and productive activity and their time.

The opportunities for productive activity outside of employment are endless; however, service providers in the fields of aging and vision-related rehabilitation need to be creative in conceptualizing and designing them. For example, opportunities for volunteer service can be informal—on a one-to-one basis, such as delivering a meal to a neighbor—or formal—through an organization such as the American Association of Retired Persons (AARP) or the Retired and Senior Volunteer Program (RSVP) (see the Resources section at the end of this module for information about these and other organizations).

It is often difficult for an older person who is visually impaired to find the right type of volunteer setting. Transportation to and from the volunteer site is always a critical consideration. Another barrier is that many people who oversee these volunteer programs think it is not possible or not safe for someone who is visually impaired to

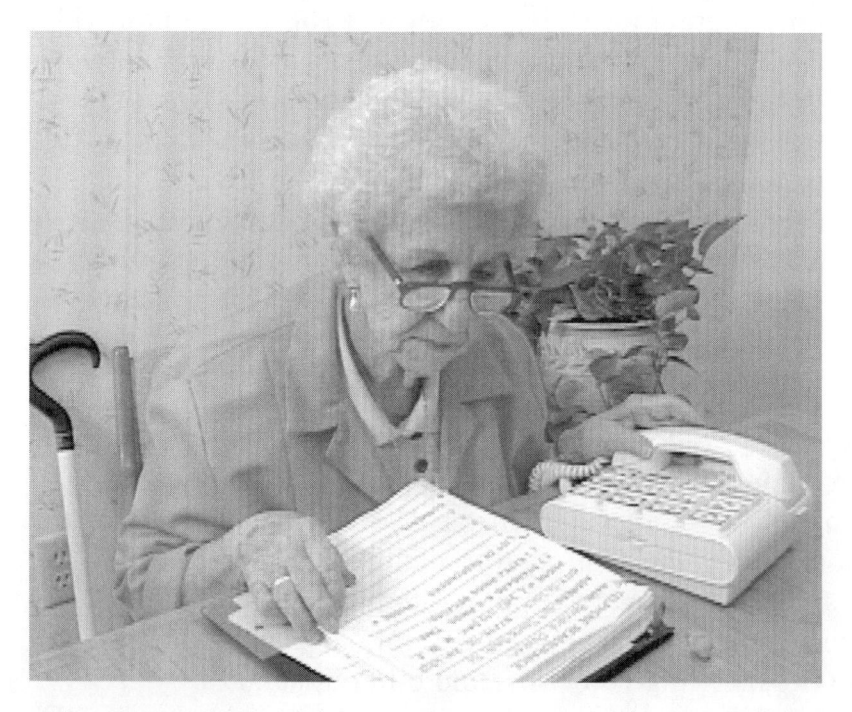

Volunteering gives older people an opportunity to use their time and skills productively and to help others in the community. This visually impaired woman volunteers to make calls to other elderly people who are confined to their homes. The large-numeral telephone and large-print directory help her in her work.

perform the task. Training these gatekeepers is key to providing such opportunities for volunteerism.

Intergenerational programs are popular and effective ways to serve both the providers and recipients of the service. They serve a variety of purposes for older persons who are visually impaired, providing opportunities for volunteerism as well as the chance to educate young people about blindness and visual impairment.

For example, older visually impaired persons involved in RSVP have served as school volunteers, addressing classes of younger people about blindness and visual impairment. Others (primarily individuals with remaining usable vision) have served as foster grandparents to young people.

Collaborative relationships between agencies serving older visually impaired persons and the agencies for the elderly that sponsor such programs facilitate meeting their clients' need for productive activity.

Leadership Roles

As noted earlier, many agencies that serve people who are blind or visually impaired are training older people who have received vision-related rehabilitation services to serve as peer counselors, peer instructors, and support group facilitators. Through these roles, older visually impaired persons have an opportunity to make a significant contribution and a difference in the lives of others. As role models for other persons experiencing age-related vision loss, they provide leadership and inspiration to their peers.

Mentoring

Mentorship is an important concept in the education and rehabilitation of individuals of any age who are blind or visually impaired. Although as a model it has thus far been underutilized in service delivery to older persons who are visually impaired, it is becoming increasingly important in educating, training, and empowering older visually impaired persons to continue to be productive, contributing members of their communities.

For example, the use of peer instructors or counselors benefits both the person serving as the role model, who feels a sense of contribution, and the other older visually impaired individual, who can be encouraged to learn new skills by witnessing the newly acquired competence and skill of the mentor.

In one national mentorship model, AFB, in cooperation with four vision rehabilitation agencies serving blind persons in different parts of the country, trained older visually impaired individuals to serve as senior companions to other older persons who were blind or visually impaired (Orr, 1992). The resulting Senior Companion Program, a federal program funded by the Corporation for National Service (formerly ACTION; see Resources), provides 20 hours per week of volunteer work for low-income older persons and provides a stipend. The visually impaired senior companions serve as models of both volunteerism and employment for older visually impaired persons. Many individuals are able to earn the additional funds they need to manage their monthly expenses.

A partnership between an agency serving blind and visually impaired persons and an agency serving elderly persons that sponsors a Senior Companion Program can be a valuable model of cooperation in improving and expanding services and opportunities for productive activity for older individuals who are visually impaired.

Although many agencies utilize the Senior Companion Program as a source of volunteers to work with their older visually impaired clients, these programs also need to consider providing opportunities for older visually impaired persons themselves to become providers of services.

6.1.9 Collaborative Models

During the 1990s, agencies serving people who are blind or visually impaired began to recognize that it is no longer possible to serve older persons with visual impairments solely within the confines of the vision rehabilitation agency. The needs of older people can be met more effectively and efficiently through cooperative and collaborative relationships and partnerships among the various service organizations and agencies within the community (see Module 7).

In addition, it is increasingly essential for agencies serving blind and visually impaired persons to function as a community resource, educating the community on many levels as well as providing services to clients. These agencies have a critical and valuable service to offer the community. They can offer training at many levels in community-based agencies and in long-term facilities.

Community education and in-service training programs are frequently the first step toward developing partnerships with agencies that serve older persons. Other types of collaborative partnerships that flow from the models of innovative service described here have already been discussed in this section. Referrals between the two systems are discussed in Module 5, and the process of building collaboration is discussed in more detail in Module 7.

6.2 Current Issues in the Vision Rehabilitation Field

As already noted, evolving conditions in society—in particular, the growing numbers of elderly people in need of vision rehabilitation and related services and the limitations in the funding of such services—require changes in the field of vision rehabilitation if it is to meet the needs of all its constituents. These circumstances necessitate not only innovative methods of service delivery such as those just discussed, but also in-depth consideration of such fundamental policy and service delivery questions as which services should be given priority based on limited funding and personnel services; who is credentialed to provide these services and under what agency auspices; and how they will be funded. This section reviews several such issues that are currently of concern to professionals in the field of vision-related rehabilitation.

6.2.1 Funding Issues

An unfortunate reality is that funding can drive service delivery. The needs of older visually impaired people will become a priority only through innovative public policy that supports increased availability of funds for the services older persons require.

As described in detail in Module 4, the grants to state rehabilitation agencies authorized by Title VII, Chapter 2 of the Rehabilitation Act—Independent Living Services for Older Individuals Who Are Blind—provide the only consistent source of funding for vision-related rehabilitation services for older individuals at present. As noted, the program not only provides essential services and trains individuals to live independently, but it is also cost-effective. The average total cost of service delivery is only $500 to $600 per person, as a result of collaborative working relationships with community agencies that "stretch" the funds. It enables older people who are visually impaired to continue to live on their own, reducing the need for more costly support services such as community-based long-term care services or nursing home care.

These funds are still very limited, however, so that all older people who are eligible are not served. Agencies are sometimes hesitant to promote the availability of independent living services or to carry out extensive outreach to unserved and underserved older people because of the lack of funds for these services. Agencies have to make optimum use of the limited funds. Thus, states with a large population of older visually impaired persons may not be able to use funds for expensive adaptive equipment, such as closed-circuit televisions (CCTVs), whereas states with fewer people in need may be able to cover these costs.

Continued legislative advocacy to preserve the Title VII, Chapter 2 program is crucial. Despite its significance, the program is at risk of being abolished or absorbed by other programs every time the Rehabilitation Act is up for reauthorization and each year when program funds are appropriated. But, although a strong program would help lift the burden from other sources of services for older persons, few professionals outside the vision rehabilitation field are aware of its existence, its benefits to older consumers, or the limited funding available to provide essential vision-related rehabilitation services. And, because the vision rehabilitation field is small in comparison to the aging network or allied health professionals, there is a strong need to broaden the advocacy base to these other groups to strengthen efforts to make sure that this federal funding continues.

Because of the limited funds available for vision rehabilitation, particularly for older people experiencing late-life onset, leaders in the vision field recognize the need to both increase and diversify the sources of funding. Among the avenues under consideration is the possibility of obtaining third-party reimbursement from the health care system for vision rehabilitation services (Lidoff, 1997).

Professionals in the vision field suggest that just as physical and occupational therapists receive such third-party reimbursement through public (Medicare and Medicaid) and private health insurance for providing rehabilitation to restore physical functioning after a hip fracture, for example, so the professionals who provide vision rehabilitation to restore independent functioning after vision loss should be eligible for reimbursement for their restorative therapeutic interventions.

6.2.2 Vision Rehabilitation Therapists

Within the vision rehabilitation field, three groups of professionals have been involved in rehabilitation of individuals with impaired vision: the rehabilitation teacher, the mobility specialist, and the low vision instructor. Recently there has been a movement toward providing services in applied settings, particularly in the homes of older adults, and this trend has called into question the need to send three different professionals to an individual's home, particularly in an era of scarce personnel and funding resources.

In addition, since impaired vision is no longer a "low incidence" phenomenon, more older persons with impaired vision are being served in a variety of settings, by a variety of professionals—for example, in health care settings, in generic rehabilitation facilities, and in long-term care facilities, in addition to their own homes. Service providers in the aging network are also seeing more clients with vision problems.

Professionals with expertise in physical rehabilitation strategies, such as occupational therapists (OTs) and physical therapists (PTs), are eager to respond to the rehabilitation needs of older adults with vision problems. Occupational therapists in particular already provide such service to this population. However, most OTs do not have specialized academic preparation, knowledge, or skills training related to vision-related rehabilitation.

To enhance the supply of highly qualified and uniquely trained professionals in vision rehabilitation who are experts certified or licensed to provide specialized vision-related rehabilitation services, the Coalition on Access to Quality Vision Rehabilitation Therapy in New York State, spearheaded by The Lighthouse, proposed that these services become the responsibility of the vision rehabilitation therapist. The recently created professional specialization of vision rehabilitation therapist combines training in the three specialized disciplines outlined: rehabilitation teaching, O&M, and low vision instruction. As a result of this proposal, a master's level personnel preparation program in vision rehabilitation has been established in New York City at Hunter College of the City University of New York.

The following benefits are anticipated from the training and proposed licensure of vision rehabilitation therapists:

- Older adults with impaired vision will be assured of receiving instruction from qualified professionals to maximize their safety and independence.
- Access to services will be increased by having the consumer work with only one professional, and the working relationship between professional and consumer will be enhanced.
- Vision rehabilitation therapists will ensure cost-effective and efficient service delivery by eliminating duplication of services.
- More multidisciplinary experts will increase the supply of qualified personnel.
- If vision rehabilitation therapists are licensed, they will be able to receive third-party reimbursement.

6.2.3 Specialized Vision-Related Services*

Another critical issue today is the preservation of specialized services for people of all ages who are blind or visually impaired. Professional and consumer organizations in the field of vision-related rehabilitation have taken the position that individuals who are blind or visually impaired, particularly older people, require specialized services, service providers, and separate agencies to meet their educational and rehabilitation needs (Spungin, 1997). The differences between generic rehabilitation services and agencies that serve exclusively people who are blind or visually impaired have a significant impact on the provision of services.

Equally important, once their specific needs related to vision loss have been met, individuals who are blind or visually impaired should have access to all other resources and services available to the general population.

Specialized programs offering training in independent living for older individuals who are blind differ from generic rehabilitation programs in several critical ways. These include personnel, programming, and data collection.

---

*This section is adapted with permission from Charles Burtis and Judy Scott, "Independent Living for Older Individuals Who Are Blind or Severely Impaired: Specialized or Generic Programming?" in J. Scott, L. Lidoff, and A. L. Orr (Eds.), *Advocacy Tools* (New York: American Foundation for the Blind, National Aging and Vision Network, February 1997).

Personnel

Vision rehabilitation professionals in agencies that serve individuals who are blind or visually impaired have specific knowledge relating to blindness, receive training in how to promote those skills needed by a person who is blind or severely visually impaired, and demonstrate techniques that are unique to teaching the older individual who is blind or severely visually impaired.

The professional staff members of generic rehabilitation programs do not receive extensive training on a specific disability but rather provide general services to people of all ages with all types of disabilities.

Programming

Although generic programs provide core independent living services, they are targeted to the general needs of people with a variety of disabilities, rather than for people with a specific and complex set of needs related to aging and vision loss. A generic program cannot concentrate on a single type of disability, such as blindness or severe visual impairment, or on a single age group. The majority of training takes place in a group setting and occurs in a separate rehabilitation facility and the primary focus is on the independent living philosophy and self-advocacy in order to obtain needed services and access to community-based resources and facilities.

In contrast, vision-related rehabilitation services provided for older individuals under the Title VII, Chapter 2 Independent Living program include hands-on training in independent living skills, orientation and mobility, braille instruction, provision of low vision aids, and community integration activities—the specific skills related to vision loss (see Module 4).

Unlike younger people who encounter disabilities, older people with significant vision loss may not have access to information about existing services or be able to access the services they need. Those who are newly visually impaired, in particular, may have difficulty at first in traveling to a rehabilitation facility and learning effectively in a setting that serves individuals with a broad range of disabilities. Individualized training in the familiar environment of an individual's own home, utilizing his or her own personal items and equipment, and rendered by a service provider who is specially trained, is critical for this population.

Data Collection

With funding of the Chapter 2 Independent Living Services for Older Individuals Who Are Blind program came not only the mandate to provide services but also a mandate to report on the numbers of individuals receiving services and the services provided (see Module 4). Each state is also required to estimate the number of individuals who qualify as potential recipients of program services.

Generic independent living services and centers are also required to make annual reports of individuals served and types of services provided. However, information on individuals who are blind or visually impaired disappears into the category labeled "sensory disability." Thus, critical data on aging and vision loss is unavailable to document the impact of services.

Such data collection is crucial and, as discussed in Module 4, needs to be expanded to include outcome measures that document the effects of these services. Reports from the agencies serving this population are also the most important source of information to document the increasing needs of older individuals who are blind or severely visually impaired—information that is essential to advocacy efforts to improve funding and services for this population.

6.2.4 Public Policy

It is crucial that funders, policymakers, the media, and all segments of the disability community be educated about the specialized interventions and services available only through the vision rehabilitation system for older individuals who are blind or severely visually impaired in order to maintain and expand services for this population. Professionals in the vision rehabilitation field need to take advantage of opportunities to influence public policy in both the aging and rehabilitation arenas that affects services to its constituency.

For example, AFB and other national organizations of and for people who are blind or visually impaired assumed active roles in bringing the issues and service needs of older persons who are blind or visually impaired to the White House Conferences on Aging in 1981 and 1995.

The National Aging and Vision Network, a national advocacy group convened by AFB consisting of professionals and consumers representing both public and private agencies that provide vision-related services to this population, has developed *Advocacy Tools*, a packet of information to assist professionals in educating policymakers and funders about the needs of older persons who are blind or visually impaired (see the Resources section at the end of the module). The Network has taken the lead in advocating to preserve and expand programs and funding for services covered under the 1997 Older Americans Act (OAA) and the Rehabilitation Act. In testimony on the reauthorization of the OAA, the Network made the following specific recommendations that would help extend the home- and community-based care provisions to older individuals who are blind or severely visually impaired (see Module 5):

Governance and Management of Home- and Community-Based Care

- Visual impairment should be included in the OAA definitions of disability and severe disability.
- Mandates should be put in place to ensure that State and Area Agencies on Aging consult and cooperate with state rehabilitation agencies which are implementing Title VII, Chapter 2 of the Rehabilitation Act (the Independent Living Services for Older Individuals Who are Blind program).
- State governments should be given the authority to ensure service funds are targeted to older persons who are most in need of support to maintain dignity and independence. This might include individuals who have recently lost their vision and who need referral to vision rehabilitation services, and/or who may need support services while waiting for receipt of such services. Often these individuals "fall between the cracks."
- States should be given the authority and flexibility to allocate Title III funds as needed to promote independent living through the provision of home- and community-based care. This would include allowing states to set functional criteria for specific home- and community-based care services.

Access to Home- and Community-Based Care

- Assessment instruments should be restructured to include questions regarding the functional abilities of individuals with severe visual impairment and the impact of vision loss on carrying out everyday tasks. (Such instruments have been developed through the network and through OAA Title IV demonstration grant monies.)
- Training on vision assessment should be provided for case managers.
- All information about home- and community-based care must be made available in alternative modes for older individuals who are

blind or visually impaired and who cannot assess printed information.

Scope of Services

- Case managers should be trained on how to refer individuals with visual impairment for vision-related rehabilitation services.
- Vision rehabilitation services such as counseling in the adjustment to vision loss, provision of adaptive aids and appliances, home modification services, and purchase of vision rehabilitation services, in the areas of mobility (travel skills) and daily living skills, should be included in home- and community-based care service packages.
- The OAA should be amended to provide funding for intergenerational programs and caregiver support. Family support is critical to the rehabilitation and continued independence of an older person who is visually impaired. Their role needs to be recognized in the Act.

Quality Improvement

- Consumer choice and customer-centered service delivery systems should be promoted in the authorization. These changes would allow states to partner more effectively with the public-private sector and to meet the expressed needs of consumers.

6.3 The Future of Service Delivery

For more than two decades, private agencies that serve blind and visually impaired persons have been reporting that a growing percentage of their clients fall into older age groups—as much as 50 percent of their caseloads. More recently, agencies are finding that 60 or 70 percent of their clients are elderly.

Service planners and providers are being challenged to develop new opportunities for sustaining valued lifelong roles; for increasing productivity, empowerment, and political activism; and for ensuring access to all needed services and resources.

The expanding population and the growing and diversifying needs of older persons who experience age-related vision loss require energy, creativity, and commitment on the part of the vision-related rehabilitation field to keep pace. The field continues to evolve, to develop innovative methods of reaching, serving, and advocating for its constituency, and to educate professionals in other fields that older visually impaired persons are part of their service delivery system as well.

Cooperative activities and networks are essential elements in the provision of comprehensive services to older visually impaired people. Agencies receiving funds under the Title VII, Chapter 2 Independent Living program have made tremendous strides in establishing collaborative partnerships with their counterparts in the field of aging to improve and expand services and to create greater access to services.

The vision-related rehabilitation field needs the service delivery and advocacy efforts of the aging network to increase funds, expand services, and create the innovative models of service delivery that will allow it to best serve the growing population of older persons experiencing vision loss. Module 7 describes collaborative partnerships among the vision field, the aging network, and other allied fields.

References

Crews, J. E., & Frey, W. D. (1993). Older people who are blind and the family members who care for them. *Journal of Visual Impairment & Blindness, 87*(1) 6–11.

A directory of self-help/mutual aid support groups for older people with impaired vision. (1994). New York: The Lighthouse.

Lidoff, L. (1997). Moving vision-related rehabilitation into the U.S. health care mainstream. *Journal of Visual Impairment & Blindness, 91*(2) 107–116.

Ludwig, I., & Schneider, P. (1991). A model of comprehensive community-based services for older blind adults. *Journal of Gerontological Social Work, 17*(3–4) 25–36.

Moore, J. E., Graves, W. H., & Patterson, J. B. (Eds.). (1997). *Foundations of rehabilitation counseling with persons who are blind or visually impaired.* New York: AFB Press.

Orr, A. L. (1992). *Visually impaired seniors as senior companions: A reference guide for program development.* New York: American Foundation for the Blind.

Spungin, S. J. (1997). A joint effort to save specialized services for adults who are blind or visually impaired. *Journal of Visual Impairment & Blindness, JVIB News Service, 91*(3), 1–6.

MODULE 6:
TRENDS AND ISSUES
IN VISION-RELATED
REHABILITATION
SERVICES

RECOMMENDED TEACHING METHODS

Lecture

Provide an overview of the current trends and issues in the delivery of vision-related rehabilitation services for older people who are blind or visually impaired.

Guest Speakers

Invite guest speakers from public or private agencies serving older blind and visually impaired persons to describe how their organizations and offices work to keep abreast of trends and issues in their field.

Small-Group Brainstorming

Organize students into small groups, and have each group brainstorm about how to build one of the innovative services discussed in this module onto a traditional service delivery model.

Field Trip

As time and resources permit, accompany students to visit an agency that has outreach services or that provides advocacy training for older people who are visually impaired. An alternative visit could be to a local business that employs older visually impaired people.

RESOURCES

Recommended Readings

Crews, J. E. (1994). Aging and disability: The issues for the 1990s. In S. E. Boone, D. Watson, & M. Bagley (Eds.), *The challenge to independence: Vision and hearing loss among older adults,* (pp. 47–60). Little Rock: University of Arkansas Rehabilitation Research and Training Center.

Kemp, B. (1994). Aging and rehabilitation: Recognizing the challenge of the older sensorially impaired person. In S. E. Boone, D. Watson, & M. Bagley (Eds.), *The challenge to independence: Vision and hearing loss among older adults* (pp. 3–14). Little Rock: University of Arkansas Rehabilitation Research and Training Center.

Lidoff, L. (1995). Home- and community-based long-term services for adults who are blind or severely visually impaired. *Journal of Visual Impairment & Blindness, 89* (6) 541–545.

Lidoff, L. (1996). Home- and community-based long-term services: Action steps. *Journal of Visual Impairment & Blindness, 90*(4), 15–16.

Lidoff, L. (1997). Moving vision-related rehabilitation into the U.S. health care mainstream. *Journal of Visual Impairment & Blindness, 91*(2), 107–116.

Orr, A. L. (1990). *Models of services delivery for older persons who are blind and visually impaired.* New York: American Foundation for the Blind.

Further Readings

Byers-Lang, R. (1984). Peer counselors, network builders for elderly blind persons. *Journal of Visual Impairment & Blindness, 78*(5), 193–197.

Byers-Lang, R., & McCall, R. (1993). Peer support groups: Rehabilitation in action. *Re:view, 25*(1), 32–36.

Cross, B. (1996). *Leadership training project, dual sensory impairment concerns: A focus on improving services.* Louisville: Kentucky Department for the Blind.

Horowitz, A., & Balistreri, E. (1994). *Field initiated research to evaluate methods for the identification and treatment of visually impaired nursing home residents.* New York: The Lighthouse.

Rogers, P. (1996). Should vision-related rehabilitation services for older persons be provided exclusively by specialists in the blindness field? *Journal of Visual Impairments & Blindness, 90*(2), 102–103.

Other Materials

A directory of self-help/mutual aid support groups for older people with impaired vision. (1994). New York: The Lighthouse.

A directory containing state-by-state listings of over 670 support groups, plus self-help clearinghouses, state agencies for the blind and visually impaired, private vision rehabilitation agencies that work with older people, national resource organizations, and a bibliography of books and articles on organizing and facilitating support groups.

Creative solutions to program needs. (1996). New York: The Lighthouse.
Lists more than 400 programs for older adults with impaired vision across the nation in the aging and vision networks. Focuses on historical development, funding, effective strategies, consumer involvement, and use of volunteers.

Orr, A. L. (1992). *Visually impaired seniors as senior companions: A reference guide for program development.* New York: American Foundation for the Blind.
A guide designed to assist service providers and others who work with blind and visually impaired older people to train, place, and match them with other older visually impaired clients so they can help each other. Describes the Senior Companion Program to help broaden opportunities for older persons with disabilities.

Orr, A. L., & Kaarlela, R. (1990). *A seven module curriculum on aging, vision loss, and independent living skills: A training model.*
A curriculum developed to train American Indians about vision rehabilitation services, which is useful in describing the role and function of the rehabilitation teacher.

Scott, J., Lidoff, L., & Orr, A. L. (Eds.). (1997). *Advocacy tools.* New York: American Foundation for the Blind, National Aging and Vision Network.
A packet of fact sheets and information about advocacy to help both consumers and professionals become advocates for vision-related rehabilitation services for older individuals who are blind or visually impaired.

Organizations

These organizations are just a few of those that can help connect older people, including those who are blind or visually impaired, to opportunities for productive activity.

American Association of Retired Persons
601 E Street, N.W.
Washington, DC 20049
(202) 434-2277

Offers a wide range of community services and educational programs, publishes a variety of pamphlets and magazines, and engages in advocacy efforts.

Corporation for National Service (formerly ACTION)
1201 New York Avenue, N.W.
Washington, DC 20525
(202) 606-5000 or (800) 424-8867
FAX: (202) 565-2789
http://www.nationalservice.org

Runs national domestic service programs, which provide opportunities to engage in community service. The National Senior Service Corps includes Foster Grandparents, Senior Companions, and the Retired and Senior Volunteer Program (RSVP).

Lighthouse National Center for Vision and Aging
11 East 59th Street
New York, NY 10022
(212) 821-9200 or (800) 334-5497 or TDD (212) 821-9713
FAX: (212) 821-9705
http://www.lighthouse.org

Serves as a national clearinghouse for information on vision and aging and referrals to services.

FACT SHEET

Integrating Older Persons Who Are Visually Impaired into a Senior Center or Other Community Activity

For many older Americans, membership and participation in a senior center is a lifeline to the community. Like other older Americans, older people who are blind or visually impaired also want to be full and active participants. There are already 5 million older persons living in communities across the country, many of whom would like to get involved in senior centers. Staff members are frequently uncertain, however, about how to make the center environment and programming accessible to those who are visually impaired. It's really not difficult. Here are some of the ways staff members or volunteers at senior centers or other community centers can help involve other people who are blind or visually impaired:

- Get in touch with a local agency that serves people who are blind or visually impaired—either the state rehabilitation agency or a local private vision rehabilitation agency. They can give you information about the special needs as well as the capabilities of older visually impaired persons.
- Have a vision rehabilitation professional from a local agency come to the center and provide in-service training for staff members on how to include visually impaired people in programs and activities.
- Arrange for training about visual impairment for senior center members with normal vision. This can make them feel more comfortable with their visually impaired counterparts and help them get involved.
- Be welcoming. When a visually impaired person joins the center, have a staff member or another senior chat with the newcomer and find out his or her interests. Establish a buddy system for orientation to the center and its programs.
- Respect the abilities of older visually impaired members. Many visually impaired seniors will want to be more than just participants. They may also want to assume leadership roles within the center. Such roles may include initiating a new center activity about which they have expertise, becoming a member of a planning committee, or joining the board of directors.

Some activities are readily accessible to older persons who are visually impaired; many others can be easily adapted. These are just a few ideas:

- Discussion groups, lectures, and oral history programs are readily accessible to visually impaired members because they are auditory.
- The local vision rehabilitation agency can give you advice about how to adapt crafts programs, dance classes, and drama and choral groups so that visually impaired members can participate.

(continued on following page)

Copyright © 1998, AFB Press

FACT SHEET

Integrating Older Persons Who Are Visually Impaired, continued

- Narration is the key to success. Visually impaired seniors can be successful at crafts, dance, and other activities, if verbal instruction is provided in addition to visual demonstration.

- When written materials are needed, such as the lines in a play or the words to the music, consult a local vision rehabilitation agency about how to get these materials in large print, braille, or on audiocassette.

Although it takes a little time and effort initially, integrating older people with disabilities—including visual impairment—can make a big difference in the overall quality of a program and in the quality of life for older persons who are blind or visually impaired.

Copyright © 1998, AFB Press

MODULE 7

Building Effective Partnerships Between the Aging Network and the Vision Rehabilitation Field

For older persons who are blind or visually impaired to receive comprehensive services and to live as independently as possible, they need both vision rehabilitation services and support services from agencies that serve elderly people. It is, therefore, vitally important that professionals in the vision rehabilitation field and aging network plan and work together on behalf of their mutual clients.

Topic Outline

7.1 The Need for Collaborative Partnerships
- **7.1.1** The Federal Level
- **7.1.2** The State Level
- **7.1.3** The Local Level

7.2 Networking Across Disciplines
- **7.2.1** Mutual Need

    7.2.2 Getting to Know Your Counterparts
    7.2.3 Local Groups on Aging
    7.2.4 In-Service Training
7.3 Developing Coalitions on Aging and Vision Loss
    7.3.1 Initiating a Coalition
    7.3.2 Membership in the Coalition
    7.3.3 Defining the Tasks of the Coalition
    7.3.4 Examples of Successful Coalitions

Learner Objectives

1. Students will be able to describe the need to collaborate across professional disciplines in order to provide comprehensive services to older individuals.
2. Students will be able to describe the steps involved in the development of a community coalition on aging and vision to address the needs of older persons who are blind or visually impaired.
3. Students will be able to list the benefits to professionals and to consumers resulting from collaborative partnerships.
4. Students will be able to list and describe four essential steps involved in effective networking.

7.1 The Need for Collaborative Partnerships

The older person who is blind or visually impaired typically needs services and assistance from both the aging network and the vision rehabilitation field as well as the health care system. Service providers need to recognize that the older visually impaired person is a mutual client of both service delivery systems and that services can be provided most effectively and efficiently through collaborative efforts between service providers in both fields.

The needs of the rapidly expanding population of older Americans, including those experiencing vision loss, place tremendous demand on the resources of both the aging network and the vision rehabilitation field. Because resources are limited, the two service

MODULE 7: BUILDING EFFECTIVE PARTNERSHIPS BETWEEN THE AGING NETWORK AND THE VISION REHABILITATION FIELD

delivery systems can benefit from working together to make the best use of existing resources, to avoid unnecessary duplication of services, and to plan ways to serve older visually impaired people most effectively.

The need for collective action between the aging network and the vision rehabilitation field through building partnerships, networking, and undertaking collaborative planning and service delivery across disciplines has been recognized for some time. Collaborative activity between the vision rehabilitation and aging fields has increased considerably since the late 1980s.

7.1.1 The Federal Level

At the federal level, the Administration on Aging (AoA) and the Rehabilitation Services Administration are the agencies representing the fields of aging and vision rehabilitation.

One model for cooperation between two federal agencies is the collaboration between the AoA and the Administration on Developmental Disabilities (both part of the Department of Health and Human Services). Starting in the late 1980s, the AoA began to recognize the need to improve services for the growing number of individuals who were developmentally disabled who were remaining in the community as they aged. The two agencies established a memorandum of understanding encouraging joint efforts to ensure access to services from the aging network for this population.

In 1994, former Assistant Secretary for Aging Fernando Torres Gil, issued a formal Information Memorandum from the AoA to State Units on Aging (SUAs) (*Fact Sheet on Title VII Chapter 2 Program of the Rehabilitation Act of 1973 as Amended*, 1994) about the Independent Living Services for Older Individuals Who Are Blind program. The memorandum sought to make service providers in the aging network aware of this program as a resource to the aging field in serving older individuals who are experiencing vision loss.

Efforts are being made by leaders in the vision rehabilitation field to create an effective partnership with the aging network at the national level, to increase understanding of the issues and service needs of older persons who are blind or visually impaired, and to facilitate more collaborative activity.

For example, in 1988, the National Council of State Agencies for the Blind reached out to the National Association of State Units on

Aging (see the Resources section at the end of this module). The two associations established a memorandum of understanding, agreeing to work collaboratively at the national and state levels for their mutual goal of achieving independence, dignity, and well-being for all the nation's older persons, including those who are blind or visually impaired. Among the joint activities proposed were public education campaigns, efforts to ensure access to services, and professional development and training.

Around the same time, the National Association of Area Agencies on Aging published an article on vision-related rehabilitation services and the Chapter 2 program with a similar goal (Lidoff, 1994).

These and similar types of information sharing at the federal level need to continue, especially as new leadership comes into office.

7.1.2 The State Level

Collaboration is especially important between the State Unit on Aging (SUA) (see Module 5) and the state vision rehabilitation agency (either a state commission for the blind or the general vocational rehabilitation agency) (see Module 4). The state level is the optimal level for agencies to plan together because SUAs are responsible for planning service delivery (whereas Area Agencies on Aging (AAAs) are responsible for carrying out plans and policies on the local level).

The state agencies for aging and vision rehabilitation are more often than not located in close proximity, frequently in the same state office building. Nevertheless, in many states the two agencies were unaware of each other until the late 1980s or 1990s. Increasingly, however, state agencies serving blind and visually impaired persons are reaching out to their counterparts in the aging field, recognizing that the two service arenas must begin to work collectively to make maximum use of limited resources.

During the 1990s, many of the Title VII, Chapter 2 project directors have established good working relationships with the corresponding SUAs and AAAs. Both formal and informal commitments have been made to work together on behalf of their mutual constituencies.

Several states have developed official memoranda of understanding at the state level that have elevated the working relationships of the two state agencies to a new level of collaboration. (A sample of such a memorandum is included in the Appendix to this chapter as a model.)

7.1.3 The Local Level

At the local level, collaboration can take place between the AAA and a local agency—the local office of the state rehabilitation agency and/or private agencies serving people who are blind or visually impaired.

Collaboration at the local level can take place through the types of coalitions on aging and vision loss described in the third section of this module. Specific examples would include the five model eldercare coalitions described in Section 7.3.4.

Local collaborative efforts are frequently the result of an innovative and creative individual—a service provider or administrator—who recognizes the need for working together to ensure access to needed services. Indeed, an important goal of this curriculum is the development of creative leadership that will foster such partnerships.

7.2 Networking Across Disciplines

7.2.1 Mutual Need

As already noted, agencies in the fields of gerontology and vision rehabilitation need each other to guarantee that they are working toward meeting all the needs of older individuals who are blind or visually impaired. Limited resources—primarily limitations in funding and personnel resources—can be powerful motivators for collective action.

7.2.2 Getting to Know Your Counterparts

Getting to know service providers in the vision rehabilitation field, as well as learning about vision rehabilitation services, eligibility criteria, and appropriate referrals to agencies serving blind and visually impaired persons, will help service providers in the aging network feel confident about working with older persons who are blind or visually impaired. Although there are many ways to effect interdisciplinary exchange, developing a formal structure such as a coalition or other group ensures better understanding among all professionals.

7.2.3 Local Groups on Aging

Providers of service to older persons in a given community typically have a local group that meets regularly to deal with issues relating to aging, such as an interagency council on aging, task force on case management, or coalition mobilizing around a particular community issue affecting older people. Inviting professionals in the vision rehabilitation field to join such groups will enhance the awareness of all involved about the specially trained professionals who provide essential services. Professionals entering the field of aging can take a leadership role in ensuring such collaborative activity.

7.2.4 In-Service Training

Service providers in the vision rehabilitation field are excellent resources for conducting training for staff members of agencies in the aging field about the needs and capabilities of elderly individuals who are blind and visually impaired. Many state and local agencies have developed in-service training programs for this purpose. Workshops on aging and vision loss for older people who use the agencies' services have also proved useful (see Module 5).

The action-oriented phrases used to describe various program initiatives of the 1990s—such as "collective action and advocacy," "strategic alliances," "partnership building," "collaborative planning and service delivery," "coalition building," and "building bridges"—indicate the significance of collaboration across many disciplines and service areas to achieve mutual goals.

7.3 Developing Coalitions on Aging and Vision Loss*

Coalitions bring together dissimilar individuals and organizations within an informal structure to work on a goal that they collectively identify. Coalitions work together in a common effort for a common purpose to make more effective and efficient use of resources. Through collective action, coalitions can have a greater impact and accomplish more than any one individual, agency, or organization.

The development of a local coalition on aging and vision loss can bring together people from many segments of the community. They can use their combined resources to develop strategies for meeting the basic daily needs of older persons experiencing age-related vision

---

*This section is adapted from "Developing a Local Coalition on Aging and Vision," by A. L. Orr, in A. L. Orr, L. Lidoff, and J. Scott (Eds.), *Building Bridges: A Resource Packet for Serving Older Visually Impaired Persons* (New York: American Foundation for the Blind, 1994).

loss who are trying to continue to live independently as well as for educating others about vision loss among the elderly population.

7.3.1 Initiating a Coalition

A coalition may be initiated by anyone in the community, but most typically is begun by an agency that serves elderly people or an agency that serves older blind and visually impaired persons. One effective method of starting a coalition is through the joint effort of both types of agencies. Through their collaborative partnership, they can reach out successfully to other segments of the community.

The overall objectives of a coalition focusing on community issues involving aging and vision would include such goals as these:

- increasing public awareness about the needs of older persons who are blind or visually impaired
- ensuring access to existing services for this population
- identifying nontraditional resources to improve the lives and independent functioning of visually impaired individuals
- ensuring access to home- and community-based services to avoid unnecessary and premature nursing home placement
- coordinating advocacy efforts with legislators and policymakers to preserve and strengthen services for older people who are experiencing age-related vision loss

Elements of effective coalitions include the following:

- skilled leadership from the coordinator
- the involvement of community leaders and various segments of the community
- clearly defined goals and objectives and courses of action to achieve them
- a defined process to achieve the coalition's mission
- goals and activities defined by the membership

7.3.2 Membership in the Coalition

A local coalition on aging and vision can draw participation from the following community arenas, all of which can provide access to services or opportunities for participation for older persons who are visually impaired:

- agencies that serve people who are blind and visually impaired
- representatives of the state agency for services to people who are blind and visually impaired

- representatives of the local AAA
- local private agencies that serve elderly persons in home- and community-based care
- local businesses such as department stores and pharmacies
- business and trade associations, including chambers of commerce
- home care organizations and hospitals
- family caregivers and family caregiver organizations
- consumer organizations of older individuals
- consumer organizations of individuals who are blind or visually impaired, such as the American Council of the Blind (ACB) and the National Federation of the Blind (NFB)
- women's organizations, such as the Older Women's League
- civic associations
- fraternal organizations, such as local Lions Clubs
- charitable and voluntary organizations
- religious institutions and organizations
- members of the clergy
- representatives of university gerontology programs
- organizations for professionals in the field of aging
- eye care professionals (ophthalmologists, optometrists, and low vision specialists)

Coalitions can energize, enable, facilitate, and empower both service providers and other leaders in the community to play a collective and active role in improving the lives of older people who are blind or visually impaired.

7.3.3 Defining the Tasks of the Coalition

As a coalition is assembled, the members themselves need to decide the particular issues and activities on which it will focus. The coalition can use the combined expertise of coalition members to

1. assess the needs of older persons who are blind or visually impaired in their local community;
2. assign priorities to these needs; and
3. determine the feasibility of addressing each priority.

Once the coalition has identified the needs it will target, the next step is to define specific strategies to address these needs.

Coalitions typically work in committees. Depending on the strategies chosen, the coalition might set up some of the following committees and activities:

- *Public Relations or Public Education:* community awareness days about aging and vision loss; development of public education materials
- *Special Projects:* in-service training sessions; one-day conferences on aging and vision loss
- *Product Development:* a directory of community services for older visually impaired persons; consumer education or consumer rights brochures
- *Legislative Advocacy:* public hearings or forums on legislative, policy, and service delivery issues

7.3.4 Examples of Successful Coalitions

A number of examples of successful coalitions on vision and aging were created through a project to improve access to services for older visually impaired persons through eldercare coalitions, initiated by the American Foundation for the Blind (AFB) and funded through AoA (Orr, Lidoff, & Scott, 1994). The overall goal of this project was to heighten the level of awareness at the community level among professionals and the general public about the needs and capabilities of older persons who are blind and visually impaired.

During the years 1992–94, AFB initiated and developed five model coalitions on aging and vision in Baltimore, Maryland; Columbia, South Carolina; Little Rock, Arkansas; Augusta, Georgia; and Huntsville, Alabama (see the Resources section at the end of this module). Each coalition assessed the needs of the older visually impaired residents in its own community through surveys, focus groups, or brainstorming sessions.

Among the key access issues identified and addressed by the coalitions were the following:

- improving access to the home- and community-based long-term care services provided through the aging network
- improving access to vision rehabilitation services
- improving access to paratransit and fixed-route transit
- creating opportunities for productive activity through involvement in the coalition and active participation in coalition activities and events
- improving access to community resources, activities, and special events not otherwise accessible to older visually impaired persons
- improving access for senior citizens' environments

- expanding opportunities for integration into senior citizens' centers, programs, or activities

The coalitions started by developing resource and public education materials in accessible formats such as large print, braille, or audiocassette. They also conducted public and professional educational activities such as workshops, conferences, and community awareness days.

Among the specific activities conducted by the various coalitions were these:

- distribution of flyers about the coalition
- insertion of information about the coalition in bank statements, utility bills, and church bulletins
- activities to heighten the level of public awareness among professionals and the general public about the issues, service needs, and capabilities of older persons who are blind or visually impaired
- identification of older persons who are blind or visually impaired who had not received vision-related rehabilitation services
- inclusion of issues about aging and vision loss on the agendas of ongoing community activities
- production of resource directories about community services and resources
- development of a "how-to" guide for family caregivers, describing independent living skills training, orientation and mobility training, communication skills, adaptive devices, tips on travel, and accessible leisure activities
- a one-day conference on Maximizing the Independence of Elderly Blind and Visually Impaired Persons for professionals in the field of aging
- a one-day community training workshop for service providers in the aging network
- a volunteer service program to assist older persons who are blind or visually impaired in their homes and in the community
- a senior citizen sporting event using sound devices and verbal cues to make the activities accessible to older participants who were blind or visually impaired
- a legislative forum on aging and vision loss that focused on policy and service delivery issues to improve access to services, attended by approximately 300 professionals and consumers from 15 states

The project's final product was the development and dissemination of *Building Bridges: A Resource Packet for Serving Older Visually Impaired Persons* (see Resources).

Ongoing activities at the end of the project included the development of accessible transportation services and descriptive video services (a service that provides additional narration to explain the visual elements occurring on the screen) for home television programs.

Within each of the five communities in which the coalitions were established, professionals in the vision rehabilitation field established close working relationships with their counterparts in the aging network as well as in other sectors of the community. These model eldercare coalitions demonstrate the potential for improving access to services and resources in the community for older persons who are blind and visually impaired through collaborative planning and collective action.

References

Administration on Aging. (1994, September). *Fact sheet on Title VII Chapter 2 program of the Rehabilitation Act of 1973 as amended, "Independent Living Services for Older Individuals Who are Blind."* Administration on Aging Information Memorandum (AoA-IM-94-06). Washington, DC: Author.

Lidoff, L. (1994, September). Resources for AAAs serving visually impaired older Americans, *Network News* (National Association of Area Agencies on Aging).

Orr, A. L., Lidoff, L., & Scott, J. (1994). *Building bridges: A resources packet on serving older visually impaired persons.* New York: American Foundation for the Blind.

RECOMMENDED TEACHING METHODS

Lecture

Provide an overview of the Module 7 content.

Group Discussion

Have students list all the possible services available to older persons along the continuum of long-term care, ranging from community-based to residential care.

Discuss where and how vision rehabilitation fits into the continuum of care.

Small-Group Brainstorming

Divide the class into small groups to develop strategies for creating partnerships among different groups within the community.

Have a representative from each small group report back to the group; create a composite list of the suggested strategies and discuss.

Role Playing

Have students conduct a mock session of a coalition that is working on how agencies can meet the needs of consumers who are blind or visually impaired.

Have students develop a memorandum of understanding based on the needs of the older consumers and the consortium of agencies.

RESOURCES

Recommended Readings

Orr, A. L. (1992). The future of collaborative planning and service delivery. In A. L. Orr (Ed.), *Vision and aging: Crossroads for service delivery* (pp. 347–357). New York: American Foundation for the Blind.

Stuen, C. (1991). Awareness of resources for visually impaired older adults among the aging network. In N. D. Weber (Ed.), *Vision and aging.* New York: Haworth Press.

Other Materials

Orr, A. L., Lidoff, L., & Scott, J. (1994). *Building bridges: A resources packet on serving older visually impaired persons.* New York: American Foundation for the Blind.

Includes the Executive Summary of a project for "Improving Access to Services for Older Visually Impaired Persons through Eldercare Coalitions"; pamphlets on *Developing a Local Coalition on Aging and Vision* and *Innovations for the Year 2000: Serving Older Americans Who Are Blind or Visually Impaired"*; and fact sheets on aging and vision.

Coalitions on Aging and Vision

For further information about some of the coalitions discussed in this module and their activities, contact the following organizations:

Alabama Division of Rehabilitative Services
407 Governors Drive
Huntsville, AL 35801
(205) 536-6621
FAX: (205) 533-1464

Lions World Services for the Blind
2811 Fair Park
Post Office Box 4055
Little Rock, AR 72214
(501) 664-7100
FAX: (501) 664-2743

Maryland Division of Vocational Rehabilitation
2301 Argonee Drive
Baltimore, MD 21218
(410) 554-3276
FAX: (410) 554-3299

South Carolina Commission for the Blind
1430 Confederate Avenue
Columbia, SC 29201
(803) 734-7520
FAX: (803) 734-7885

Organizations

The organizations listed here are involved in collaboration efforts with the vision rehabilitation field at the national level, and can also help identify the appropriate agencies for collaboration at the state and local levels.

National Association of Area Agencies on Aging
1112 16th Street, N.W., Suite 100
Washington, DC 20036

(202) 296-8130
FAX: (202) 296-8134
E-mail: jjfn4a@erols.com

Advocates at the national level for the needs of older persons. Disseminates information to the federal government, other national organizations, and the public. Provides referrals to local agencies and publishes an annual *Directory of State and Area Agencies on Aging.*

National Association of State Units on Aging
1225 I Street, N.W., Suite 725
Washington, DC 20005
(202) 898-2578
FAX: (202) 898-2583
E-mail: staff@nasua.org

Provides information on state services to older persons and advocates for legislation and funding for such services.

National Council of State Agencies for the Blind
1213 29th Street, N.W.
Washington, DC 20007
(202) 298-8468
FAX: (202) 333-5881

Promotes communication among agencies involved in preventing blindness and offering services to severely visually impaired individuals.

APPENDIX

Sample Memorandum of Agreement Between the Department for the Blind and the Division of Aging Services, Department of Social Services

Introduction

According to the U.S. Census data, in 1990 there were 465,000 persons age 65 or older in the state, and projections show an increase of 41 percent to 656,000 by the year 2020. Among individuals 65 and older, severe visual impairment is the third leading cause of disabilities. About 30 percent of nursing home residents are severely visually impaired.

[Additional state data can be added here].

Furthermore, published studies on older persons who are blind or visually impaired reveal the following facts about these persons.

- Existing programs and services do not reach a majority of eligible recipients.
- They lack education and knowledge about their disabilities.
- Professional eye care services, especially low vision services, are not available in many of their communities.
- They are in need of transportation to access services.
- They do not have adequate resources to pay for medical treatment and services.
- They are socially isolated from society.
- They lack knowledge and understanding of preventive measures.
- Vision rehabilitation services can reduce their dependency.

The purpose of this Memorandum of Agreement is to provide a vehicle for the Department for the Blind and its service delivery network and the Division of Aging Services, Department of Social Services and its service delivery network to expand and enhance services to a growing client population and to develop and implement a model system for providing high-quality services to an increasing number of older citizens.

This agreement states the intentions of the two agencies to establish a higher level of trust and cooperation.

WHEREAS, the Department for the Blind is the state agency designated to serve people who are blind or severely visually impaired;

WHEREAS, the Department of Social Services is the state agency designated to provide social and supportive services to needy persons;

WHEREAS, the Division of Aging Services is the single organization designated to serve older persons, and the Division of Aging Services and its contract agencies, the Area Development Districts, administer the Older American Act Programs, the Homecare Program, the Adult Day Care Programs and other programs that provide a continuum of care for older persons;

WHEREAS, the Long-Term Care Ombudsman Program is the Office mandated to serve as an advocate for the elderly in Long-Term Care settings;

WHEREAS, the Division of Family Services, Adult Services Branch, is responsible to provide or arrange supportive, protective or placement services for eligible adults;

THEREFORE, the Department for the Blind and the Division of Aging, Department of Social Services agree to the following working agreement.

1. At the State Office level, each agency will appoint liaison persons to ensure the implementation of this agreement,
2. Both agencies agree to participate in the following activities:
    a. Develop training materials and provide training for Area Agencies on Aging staff, case managers, Department for Social Services staff, Department for the Blind staff, service providers, peer support, family caregivers, and volunteers
    b. Develop and implement Aging/Vision rehabilitation internal and external outreach plans
    c. Develop or revise existing comprehensive client assessment protocols to incorporate questions about the impact of blindness and visual impairment
3. Both agencies will provide services to consumers to the extent possible with resources available.

4. Since both agencies are subject to similar regulations on confidentiality, each has the responsibility to ensure that information be shared in the interest of clients, subject to their limitations.

5. Both agencies are committed to exploring the use of other resources, such as Medicaid waiver, and demonstration grants, to continue existing services and to expand services that have proven to be successful.

FURTHER, both agencies will view this memorandum of agreement as an incentive to foster statewide cooperation and collaboration where feasible between the aging and vision rehabilitation networks.

This agreement is effective as of the _____ day of _____ the year _____ by and between the Department for the Blind and the Division of Aging and will be reviewed annually by both parties.

_____ _____
Director   Director
Division of Aging Services   Division of Client Services
Department for Social Services Department for the Blind

_____ _____
Commissioner   Commissioner
Department for Social Services Department for the Blind

_____ _____
Attorney (as needed)   Attorney (as needed)

Glossary

Accommodation The ability of the eye to alter its focus to see objects at various distances by changing the shape of the lens.

Activities of daily living (ADL) The routine activities that an individual must be able to perform in order to live independently, such as bathing, eating, dressing, toileting, transferring from bed to a chair, and moving around the house.

Acuity See Visual acuity.

Adapted device An object, such as a talking clock or a large-print kitchen timer, that has been altered to help a visually impaired individual with communication, the activities of daily living, and other activities.

Adaptive skill A technique or method that helps a visually impaired individual with communication, the activities of daily living, or other activities.

Adventitious Occurring after birth; not present at birth. With regard to a visual impairment, it also means occurring after early childhood dvelopmental stages are complete.

Age-related macular degeneration (ARMD) A degenerative disease of the macula that causes loss of central vision, resulting in a central scotoma, or a blind or partially blind area in the central visual field; one of the most common visual impairments in elderly people. Also called age-related maculopathy.

Amsler grid A graphlike card used to determine central field losses, as in macular degeneration.

Aqueous The clear fluid in the space between the vitreous and the back of the cornea, produced by the ciliary processes, that bathes the lens and nourishes the iris

GLOSSARY

and inner surface of the cornea. Also called aqueous humor.

Area Agency on Aging The agency designated by federal legislation to serve as a focal point for programs and services to older people within a local planning and service area.

Assessment In vision rehabilitation, the process through which the vision rehabilitation professional determines the present needs and skill levels of the client.

Binocular vision The ability to use two eyes together to focus on the same object by fusing two images into one.

Blindness Lack of functional vision.

Braille A tactile system for reading and writing, based on a cell composed of six raised dots.

Cataracts A clouding of the lens of the eye, which may be congenital, traumatic, secondary to another visual impairment, or age-related.

CCTV See Closed-circuit television.

Central vision The perception of images focused on the central area of the retina (macula); used to identify and obtain detailed information about objects.

Closed-angle glaucoma A form of primary glaucoma characterized by an increase in intraocular pressure as a result of a blockage of the anterior chamber at the base of the iris. Closed-angle glaucoma can cause sudden vision loss and immediate pain. Also called narrow-angle glaucoma.

Closed-circuit television (CCTV) A device, used primarily as a reading aid for persons with low vision, that electronically magnifies printed material by means of a camera and projects the enlarged image on a video monitor.

Cones Specialized photoreceptor cells in the retina, primarily concentrated in the macular area, that are responsible for sharp vision and color perception.

Congenital Present at birth; in the case of blindness or visual impairment, occurring at birth or before early childhood development.

Contrast Dissimilarity in color of adjacent parts; providing appropriate contrast for tasks improves the visual performance of individuals with low vision.

Contrast sensitivity The ability to detect differences in grayness and background.

Convergence The movement of both eyes toward each other as an object approaches, in an effort to maintain fusion of separate images.

Depth perception The overlapping of two slightly dissimilar images from the two eyes to perceive the relative positions of objects in the visual field, giving three-dimensional vision.

Diabetic retinopathy A complication of diabetes mellitus stemming from changes in the retinal blood vessels, characterized by retinal hemorrhages, neovascularization, and scarring; a leading cause of blindness in the United States.

Distance vision The ability to see objects from a distance; distance visual acuity is measured using distance vision test charts such as the Snellen chart.

Drusen The yellow spots of waste material that appear on the retina; drusen are a symptom of "dry" acute macular degeneration.

Eccentric viewing An adaptive low vision skill that involves shifting the gaze to use the functioning areas of the retina when a scotoma interferes with a person's ability to see objects in the central field.

Electronic magnification systems Equipment that produces enlarged images, including closed-circuit televisions, computer systems, and low vision enhancement devices.

Field See Visual field.

Field loss A measure of deficiency of vision based on what a fixed eye can or cannot see; it may be either peripheral or central vision loss.

Fixation The ability of the eyes to direct and hold the gaze on an object to enable an image to focus on the retina.

Floaters Deposits or particles in the vitreous that appear as thin, transparent strings or specks that flutter and float through the visual field; a sudden appearance of floaters or flashes of light may indicate a serious eye disorder, such as a retinal tear.

Fovea An indentation in the center of the macula where the cones are concentrated, there are no blood vessels, and the clearest vision takes place.

Functional vision The ability to use vision in planning and performing a task.

Glare An annoying sensation produced by too much light in the visual field that can cause both discomfort and a reduction in visual acuity.

Glaucoma A condition characterized by an increase in intraocular pressure, associated with a buildup of aqueous fluid, that may cause damage to the nerves of the retina and the optic nerve and eventual loss of visual field if left untreated.

Hemianopia A defect in either half of the visual field. Also called hemianopsia.

Home- and community-based care (HCBC) A program that offers a full range of services and settings to elderly or disabled people to enable them to continue living in their own homes or in a residential care setting in the community.

Incidence The number or percentage of new occurrences of a patrticular condition in a population in a given time period, typically a year.

Instrumental activities of daily living Essential activities required for an individual to be able to carry out the basic activities of daily living, such as shopping for and preparing food in order to consume food; also doing housework, managing money, using the telephone, managing medication, walking outside, using public transit, and the like.

Large print (large type) Print that is larger (18 points or more) than that commonly found in magazines, newspapers, and books (6–12 points).

Legal blindness Visual impairment in which distance visual acuity is 20/200 or less in the better eye after best correction with conventional lenses, or a visual field restriction of 20 degrees or less; often used as a criterion for determining eligibility for benefits or services in the United States.

Lens The transparent biconvex structure (disk) within the eye, located behind the iris, that allows it to refract light rays, enabling the rays to focus on the retina; also called the crystalline lens.

Light perception The ability to discern the presence or absence of light, but not its source or direction.

Low vision A degree of vision that is functional but limited enough to interfere with the ability to perform everyday activities and that cannot be corrected with standard eyeglasses or contact lenses.

Low vision assessment A comprehensive appraisal of a visually impaired individual's visual impairment, visual potential, and visual ability to determine whether the person can benefit from optical devices, nonoptical devices, or adaptive techniques to enhance visual function.

Low vision devices Various types of optical and nonoptical devices used to enhance the visual capability of persons with visual impairments. See also Nonoptical and Optical devices.

Low vision specialist An ophthalmologist or optometrist who specializes in low vision care.

Macula The central area of the retina, which is the area of best visual acuity and is responsible for fine near-vision tasks such as reading and sewing.

Macular degeneration See Age-related macular degeneration.

Magnifier A low vision device used for short-term near-vision spotting tasks that can increase the size of an image on the retina through the use of lenses and may have either a fixed focus (such as a stand magnifier) or a variable focus (such as a handheld magnifier).

Microscope A low vision device, used for near-vision tasks, that uses magnification.

Neuropathy An abnormal and usually degenerative state of the nervous system or nerves, as in the reduced tactile sensitivity in diabetic neuropathy.

Nonoptical device A device that does not involve optics, used to make visual information and visual functioning more accessible to individuals with low vision, such as a writing guide, large-print telephone keypad, book stand, or high-intensity lamp.

Open-angle glaucoma The most common type of primary glaucoma, in which the aqueous humor does not filter through the trabecular meshwork and out of the Canal of Schlemm; it is bilateral and asymptomatic in onset until visual impairment occurs, and then is slowly progressive. See also Glaucoma.

Ophthalmologist A physician who specializes in the medical and surgical care of the eyes and is qualified to prescribe ocular medications and to perform surgery on the eyes. May also perform refractive and low vision work, including eye examinations and other vision services.

Optical device A low vision device that incorporates optics, such as a magnifier, microscope, or telescope.

Optics The science that deals with light and phenomena associated with it, applied in the prescription of low vision devices.

Optometrist A health care provider who specializes in refractive errors, prescribes eyeglasses or contact lenses, and diagnoses and manages conditions of the eye as regulated by state law.

Orientation and mobility (O&M) The vision rehabilitation field dealing with systematic techniques by which blind or visually impaired persons orient themselves to their environment and move about independently.

Orientation and mobility (O&M) instructor A professional who specializes in teaching travel skills to visually impaired persons, including the use of a cane, dog guide, or sophisticated electronic travel aids, as well as the sighted guide technique.

Peripheral vision The ability to perceive the presence, motion, or color of objects outside the direct line of vision or by other than the central retina.

Photophobia Light sensitivity to an uncomfortable degree; usually symptomatic of other ocular disorders and diseases.

Photoreceptor cells Retinal cells (rods and cones) that convert light to electrical impulses that can be transmitted to the brain.

Presbyopia A decrease in accommodative power (focusing at near distance) caused by the increasing inelasticity of the lens-ciliary muscle mechanism that tends to occur anytime after age 40.

Prevalence The number or percentage of a population that is affected by a particular condition at a given time.

Pupil The hole in the center of the iris through which light rays enter the back of the eye.

Radio reading service An auditory information resource, usually operating on unused bands of radio frequencies and requiring a special receiver, that provides persons with visual, physical, and reading disabilities with information such as newspaper articles, commentary, advertisements, bestsellers not available in adapted forms, consumer information, and information on issues such as jobs, access, and transportation.

Reading machine A computer-based assistive device that converts printed text into speech.

Rehabilitation teacher A professional who provides instruction and guidance in adaptive skills to adults with visual impairments in five broad skill areas—home management, personal management, communication, indoor environmental orientation, and leisure activity—to enable the individual to live and function independently.

Retina The innermost layer of the eye, containing light-sensitive nerve cells and fibers connecting with the brain through the optic nerve that receives the image formed by the lens.

Rods Specialized retinal photoreceptor cells, located primarily in the peripheral retina, that are responsible for seeing form, shape, and movement and function best in low levels of illumination.

Scanner A device that uses a moving electronic beam to convert visual images, such as printed text or images, into an electronic format that can be transmitted or converted into other formats.

Scotoma A gap or blind spot in the visual field that may be caused by damage to the retina or visual pathways. Each eye has one normal scotoma, corresponding to the location of the optic nerve head, which contains no photoreceptors.

Screen-magnification system A computer-based system that electronically enlarges the characters displayed on a computer monitor; it may work through software only, hardware only, or combinations of both. Also known as screen-enlargement system.

Severe visual impairment As defined by the National Center for Health Statistics, the inability to read ordinary newspaper print even with the aid of corrective lenses.

State Unit on Aging The agency of a state government designated to be the focus for programs and services for older people at the state level, mandated by federal legislation.

Stereopsis Three-dimensional vision as a result of binocular fusion.

Talking Book program A free national library program administered by the National Library Service for the Blind and Physically Handicapped (NLS) of the Library of Congress for persons with visual and physical limitations, in which the books and magazines are produced in braille and on recorded discs and cassettes and are distributed to a cooperative network of regional libraries that circulate them to eligible borrowers; the program also lends the devices on which the recordings are played.

Telescope A low vision device that uses magnification for viewing objects at distances of about 2 feet or greater.

Tonometry The measurement of intraocular pressure, used to detect signs of glaucoma.

Vision rehabilitation services The full range of clinical and instructional services related to the adjustment to vision loss and the prescription and use of optical and nonoptical devices to maximize vision.

Visual acuity The sharpness of vision with respect to the ability to distinguish detail, often measured by the eye's ability to distinguish the details and shapes of objects at a designated distance; it involves central (macular) vision.

Visual field The area that can be seen when looking straight ahead, measured in degrees from the fixation point.

Visual impairment Any degree of vision loss, including total blindness, that affects an individual's ability to perform the tasks of daily life.

Visual perception The process of attaching meaning to a visual image.

Vitrectomy The surgical removal of the vitreous and its replacement with a saline solution.

Vitreous A transparent, jelly-like substance that fills the back portion of the eye between the lens and the retina and maintains the shape of the eyeball.

Vocational rehabilitation The process of preparing an individual for useful employment by means of evaluation, vocational counseling, and training in job skills in preparation for optimal placement.

Writing guide An adaptive device that assists a visually impaired individual in determining the space in which to write or in writing on a line.

About the Author

Alberta L. Orr is the chair of the National Aging Program of the American Foundation for the Blind (AFB); convener of the National Aging and Vision Network, headquartered at AFB; and chair of the Aging Division of the Association for Education and Rehabilitation of the Blind and Visually Impaired. She is also the co-chair of AFB's annual Josephine L. Taylor Leadership Institute and an adjunct faculty member at Hunter College of the City University of New York where she teaches in the Rehabilitation Teaching Master's Degree Program, Department of Special Education. She has served as the principal investigator of many federally funded projects and is the author of numerous publications, including *Vision and Aging: Crossroads for Service Delivery*. She is a sought-after speaker and national leader in the field of vision and aging.

Photo and Figure Credits

American Foundation for the Blind, 44, 45, 47, 48, 60, 61, 121, 128, 180; Lighthouse Low Vision Products, 59; Pinellas Center for the Visually Impaired, 58, 63; Prevent Blindness America, 40.

The mission of the American Foundation for the Blind (AFB) is to enable persons who are blind or visually impaired to achieve equality of access and opportunity that will ensure freedom of choice in their lives.

∞

It is the policy of the American Foundation for the Blind to use in the first printing of its books acid-free paper that meets the ANSI Z39.48 Standard. The infinity symbol that appears above indicates that the paper in this printing meets that standard.